Emergency Birth
in the Community

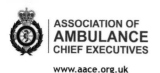

ASSOCIATION OF
AMBULANCE
CHIEF EXECUTIVES

www.aace.org.uk

jrcalc
joint royal colleges ambulance
liaison committee

www.jrcalc.org.uk

Emergency Birth in the Community

Edited for JRCALC and AACE by
Amanda Mansfield, Midwife

Disclaimer

The Association of Ambulance Chief Executives and the Joint Royal Colleges Ambulance Liaison Committee have made every effort to ensure that the information, tables, drawings and diagrams contained in these guidelines are accurate at the time of publication. However, the guidelines are advisory and have been developed to assist healthcare professionals and patients, to make decisions about the management of the patients' health, including treatments. This advice is intended to support the decision-making process and is not a substitute for sound clinical judgement. The guidelines cannot always contain all the information necessary for determining appropriate care and cannot address all individual situations; therefore, individuals using these guidelines must ensure they have the appropriate knowledge and skills to enable suitable interpretation.

The Association of Ambulance Chief Executives and the Joint Royal Colleges Ambulance Liaison Committee do not guarantee, and accept no legal liability of whatever nature arising from or connected to, the accuracy, reliability, currency or completeness of the content of these guidelines.

The information presented in this book is accurate and current to the best of the authors' knowledge. The authors and publisher, however, make no guarantee as to, and assume no responsibility for, the correctness, sufficiency or completeness of such information or recommendation.

Printing history

First published 2018

The authors and publisher welcome feedback from the users of this book.

Please contact the publisher:

Class Professional Publishing,
The Exchange, Express Park, Bristol Road, Bridgwater TA6 4RR
Telephone: 01278 427 800
Email: icpg@class.co.uk
Website: www.classprofessional.co.uk

Class Professional Publishing is an imprint of Class Publishing Ltd

A CIP catalogue record for this book is available from the British Library

This edition: Emergency Birth in the Community ISBN 9781859596814

Also available: Emergency Birth in the Community (eBook) ISBN 9781859596821

Printed in the UK by Hobbs

Typeset by S4Carlisle Publishing Services

Contents

Contents

List of Figures and Tables

List of Figures and Tables

Foreword

Pregnancy and childbirth birth is a joyous time for most families, and indeed the United Kingdom is one of the safest places to have a baby in the world. While modern antenatal care concentrates on prevention, screening and early detection of the signs of potential obstetric emergencies, it is an unavoidable fact, as in any area of medicine, that emergencies do happen.

Within this book is an exceptional level of detail describing how the physiology of a pregnant woman differs in several key ways from her non-pregnant state. By simply having a clear understanding of these differences and applying this knowledge when managing women (at all stages of pregnancy), attending responders are highly likely to help save lives in the community.

Unplanned community birth is an uncommon event. However, the summarised steps provided in this manual not only describe a practical approach to normal labour and delivery but prioritise maternal safety and ensure the immediate wellbeing of the newborn baby while awaiting transfer. The book covers simple steps employed by midwifery and obstetric staff hundreds of times a day around the world. These include my two personal favourite lifesaving actions, used many times over my career, and straightforward steps that anyone can follow:

● For a woman experiencing a post-partum haemorrhage, bleeding can often be controlled by palpating the uterus abdominally and massaging a contraction to commence a natural tamponade.

Foreword

- Once born, ensure the baby is immediately dried, wrapped and kept warm. If the mother is well, then simply place the baby in close contact with her skin. This not only helps with bonding but prevents early onset neonatal hypothermia and hypoglycaemia, both much more serious in babies born pre-term.

Safe delivery of maternity care in the UK depends on efficient and well-practised teams that have high standards of knowledge and skill. Responding in the community undoubtedly requires a different skill set, but what unites both community and hospital teams is the need for optimal communication and teamwork. What particularly stands out in this book is not only the emphasis on what to do in emergency situations but also who to involve and the most relevant messages to send to them, while still delivering the highest standards of care.

In this resource, JRCALC provides the key facts to underpin your knowledge of emergency maternity care. In addition the book includes illustrated flowcharts and other tools that are intended for top-up knowledge or to be readily available for the management of specific emergencies.

This is not just a book; it is a practical, efficient tool to help you deliver safe maternity care in the community and it has a place not only on your bookshelf but also in your back pocket.

Mr Edward Morris MD FRCOG, Vice President, Clinical Quality, Royal College of Obstetricians and Gynaecologists

Acknowledgements

As a practising midwife for over 25 years, attending out of hospital maternity emergencies continues to be one of the greatest challenges I face. For each woman, the experience of the care she receives is as important as the birth she anticipated in the calm environment of her planned place of birth. While not all events are positive and can have long-lasting effects on the woman, her family and the staff involved, it has been my intention to provide a raised awareness of the challenges responders are presented with when attending this type of emergency. I would like to thank two very special friends who have acted as my 'fresh eyes' to kindly review and add their expertise to the book: Kim Hinshaw, who has patiently provided his 'obstetric' view on this discipline and contributed his thoughts; and Aimee Yarrington, who brings her unique view as both a paramedic and a midwife.

Introduction

Birth is a unique time of life for a woman and her family, and for the majority of women it will take place in a planned environment such as her home, a birth centre or a hospital-based facility with her chosen birth partners.

While in the UK environment maternity care is provided by midwives and obstetricians (including some general practitioners or 'GPs'), in other healthcare systems, the lead professional may be someone from a range of clinician roles, including obstetric nurses and physicians.

On occasion, birth takes place unexpectedly and unplanned outside of these environments, for the following reasons:
- premature birth (less than 36/37 weeks of pregnancy);
- a very rapid (precipitous) labour, which does not provide enough time for a health professional to reach the woman, or the woman to access her chosen place of birth;
- the woman is sent home from hospital following a labour assessment, and labour progresses rapidly; or
- concealed or unknown pregnancy.

For any member of the healthcare/emergency care community (referred to here as a responder), attending a birth without previous knowledge or skills can be extremely challenging. For the woman, the attendance of a responder in an emergency may afford her a sense of safety and a perception that the individual has the requisite knowledge and skills to support birth under the circumstances.

Emergency birth is not without its challenges for the unfamiliar and inexperienced responder. The following text aims to equip and inform the reader in these challenges, through the use of informal chapters providing an oversight of each aspect of maternity care, with a section that can be used in real-time for emergency birthing situations.

This book is aimed at all staff in the community setting who may respond to emergency birth. This includes those who respond from the traditional emergency services setting (i.e. ambulance staff) as well as joint response units (e.g. fire services, police and first responders). It will equally be useful to established doctors, nurses and those operating in different health environments, who may attend with very little knowledge and/or equipment.

Early consideration should always be given to the availability of a dedicated pre-hospital team. This will be configured according to the local health system. Some areas will have the ability to undertake advanced interventions including providing critical care stabilisation, additional medical support and, on rare occasions, peri-mortem caesarean section. In some areas, midwives who can get to the emergency within a reasonable time period may be available to afford on-scene assistance.

Emergency birth occurs across all communities, including those that vary by geography and access to a nearby hospital with maternity facilities. While rural and remote settings may necessitate longer distances and longer travel times, modern built-up city areas pose different challenges in terms of access and travel times due to congestion.

Communication is a critical part of care when managing emergency birth. The importance of 'pre-arrival information' is emphasised within the book, to enable readiness of the awaiting clinical team when responders arrive with a woman and her baby. Good communication ensures that, where appropriate, particular emergencies are highlighted simply and effectively.

Introduction

Due to the variation in healthcare set up around the world, the fundamentals of the book are based upon the UK system, and these are reflected in the flow charts for use in an emergency. These can be adapted for local use where necessary.

While those professionals who are responsible for providing maternity care to a woman will be exposed to regular training to manage maternity emergencies, the typical responder may not have access to this, and it is recommended that alongside this book the healthcare system identifies the level of training to offer, dependent upon the frequency at which the emergency arises.

The book forms three distinct sections:
1. Overview of maternity emergencies before, during and after birth.
2. Emergency cards for real-time use in an emergency, to be kept within a trouser pocket or an emergency birth pack stored in the responder's kit.
3. A sample template for recording key information following an emergency birth.

Chapter 1
Maternity Care

Any woman of childbearing age may be pregnant, and, unless there is a history of hysterectomy, there must be a high index of suspicion that any abdominal pain or vaginal bleeding may be pregnancy related.

If a woman has booked for maternity care, she should have access to her hand-held records (these may be electronic, or in the form of a paper book) or be able to provide details of her care provider. Within her maternity records, a detailed history will include key information to help those that are attending, including:
- relevant history regarding the current pregnancy (if known) and any previous pregnancies;
- relevant medical history;
- emergency contact details (this may be the partner, family member or a friend); and
- if the woman is booked for maternity care, the name of the lead clinician (may be a midwife, obstetrician or obstetric nurse) or the name of the maternity unit providing maternity care.

When attending an emergency birth, it is important to be aware of the impact of both the environment and the situation upon your decision making. Being aware of where you are and how to maintain a safe environment while supporting the woman, are both key to ensuring a safe outcome.

There may be other people attending who are related or known to the woman and/or bystanders, who are able to assist. The birth may be taking place in a public area, such as a train station or a supermarket, where ensuring the privacy and dignity of the woman and the baby at this intimate time are crucial.

Working as a team at an emergency birth is key to a successful outcome for mother and newborn baby. While others in attendance may not be health professionals or responders, delegating tasks and clear communication can ensure that the birth will be calm for the woman, while enabling each person to work well together and provide a positive experience for everyone involved.

Factors that can affect our behaviour in an emergency include teamwork, tasks, equipment and the work environment. Knowledge of these and their impact on clinical performance can enable an understanding of our behaviour in this setting.

Lines of communication between individuals should promote the ability to share, through verbal communication, an agreed 'plan' or shared 'mental model' of what the team is doing and what the team is planning. An understanding of human factors and situational awareness equips responders with enhanced clinical performance and safe practice.

The responder should consider early involvement with pre-hospital medical and midwifery teams where available.

There are a very limited number of drugs that are required during an emergency birth. These will be clearly defined within the scope of the responder. In the UK, common drugs include the following:

Pain relief
Entonox (nitrous oxide and oxygen): inhalational pain relief, rapidly absorbed and excreted, commonly carried by midwives, ambulance clinicians (paramedics and doctors) and some responders.

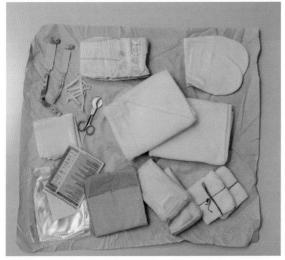

Figure 1.1 *A typical maternity pack used by a UK NHS Ambulance Trust.*

Uterotonics used for the management of post-partum haemorrhage

Syntometrine (Oxytocin 5 IU and Ergometrine 500 micrograms in 1ml ampoule) may be used in the absence of hypertension. Intramuscular injection to stimulate uterine contraction and control bleeding after the birth of the baby. Commonly carried by midwives, ambulance clinicians and pre-hospital medical teams.

● Syntocinon (Oxytocin 5 or 10 IU) can be given if the mother has a history of hypertension or pre-eclampsia. Intramuscular injection to stimulate uterine contraction and control bleeding after the birth of the baby.

- Misoprostol 800 micrograms may be given if the above uterotonic drugs are unavailable. Used to stimulate uterine contraction. Given sublingually, unless the patient is unable to maintain their airway and the rectal route may be considered appropriate.

Management of Convulsions
- Diazepam or Magnesium Sulphate: intravenous injection to control fitting associated with either epilepsy or eclampsia after 20 weeks of pregnancy.

Each local area will have identified what maternity kit or equipment responders have access to. Key components should include the following (see Figure 1.1):
- two towels: one to dry the baby, the other to wrap the baby with its skin directly on the mother's skin to optimise the temperature of the baby;
- one or two newborn hats to reduce heat loss, due to the large surface area of the baby's head in relation to its body;
- a nappy: the woman may have a nappy available, but one should be available in the kit to absorb urine and/or meconium, and avoid the newborn losing heat if surround by wet fluids.
- a bag, which can be used to store the placenta and membranes until they can be inspected for completeness. Some women and their families want to keep the placenta. It is therefore important to ask the woman for her consent to remove and dispose of the placenta.
- two plastic clamps: one to clamp the maternal end of the cord following the birth of the placenta, the other near the newborn abdomen (note that it is not necessary to clamp the cord immediately after birth); and
- a set of sterile scissors to cut the umbilical cord once it has stopped pulsating or the placenta has birthed.

Other items of value include sanitary towels and x-ray detectable gauze swabs, for application of external pressure to any perineal trauma that is actively bleeding.

Appropriate Destination for Conveyance

The choice of destination to convey a mother and/or her baby/babies should be carefully considered and in line with agreed local policies depending upon the maternal healthcare system. Consideration should always be given to where the nearest appropriate facility is located. A pregnant woman will have been given a choice of where to birth her baby: at her home, a standalone birth centre (which may be remotely located from the main obstetric unit), a birthing centre within a maternity unit, on a labour ward or in a delivery suite. It is key to ensure that local pathways clearly identify which facilities are available in the event of an emergency birth or maternity emergency.

Local networks may vary in the level of obstetric and neonatal facilities present and this should be considered in the local arrangements for this type of emergency planning.

If a woman has planned her care at a particular unit and this is not the nearest facility, in an emergency situation this may have to be overridden.

The nearest emergency department (ED) will be the appropriate destination when there is a cardiac arrest, major airway problems or ongoing eclamptic convulsions and severe uncontrolled bleeding. Those EDs that have an obstetric facility are preferable for patients with ongoing eclamptic convulsions and severe uncontrolled bleeding. The priority is always to stabilise the critical condition of the patient, a secondary transfer can then be undertaken.

In other obstetric emergencies (e.g. shoulder dystocia, mild to moderate bleeding etc.) transfer to the nearest full obstetric unit (i.e. not a birthing centre or 'standalone' midwifery unit) will be appropriate. Remember that in many cases, a full obstetric unit will be co-located with an ED, but this may not always be the case.

Careful consideration should always be given to the most appropriate destination in each case. Also consider carefully the accessibility of a unit (e.g. out-of-hours, locked doors, corridors and lifts). In line with local procedures, pre-alert arrangements and telephone numbers should be agreed and readily available.

Key Points for Maternity Care

- Any woman of childbearing age may be pregnant.
- Working as a team at an emergency birth is key to a successful outcome for the mother and newborn baby.
- The choice of destination to convey a mother and/or her baby or babies should be carefully considered and in line with agreed local policies depending upon the maternal healthcare system.

Chapter 2

Assessment of the Pregnant Woman

Pregnancy is timed from the first day of the last period and may last up to or in excess of 42 weeks. The pregnancy is divided into three trimesters (1–12 weeks + 6 days, 13–25 weeks + 6 days and 26 weeks +). A pregnancy is defined as being at 'term' if the number of weeks of pregnancy are greater than 37 completed weeks. A baby born at less than this gestation may require additional medical support, which is detailed in Chapter 5. Therefore, knowing the gestation of the pregnancy is key to anticipating the potential challenges you may be presented with.

If the woman does not know how many weeks pregnant she is, or a language barrier is present, a visual inspection of the highest point of the uterus (fundal height) can normally guide the responder. If the fundal height is at the level of the woman's umbilicus, the gestation of the pregnancy equates to roughly 22 weeks and suggests that if the unborn baby (fetus) is born, it may not survive due to its prematurity.

There are a multitude of physiological and anatomical changes during pregnancy that may influence the assessment and management of the pregnant woman.

Cardiovascular changes:
- Increase in cardiac output by 20–30% by 10 weeks of pregnancy.
- Average increase in maternal heart rate by 10–15 bpm.
- Reduction in blood pressure by an average of 10–15 mmHg.

- From 20 weeks onwards, the pregnant uterus may cause compression on the inferior vena cava, reducing venous return, and lowering cardiac output by 40% when the woman lies on her back (supine), which can in turn reduce her blood pressure. Positioning the patient either on her left side, or manual uterine displacement to the maternal left, will reduce the pressure on the inferior vena cava and improve cardiac stability.
- The combined effect of the pregnant uterus, and the reduction in peripheral vascular resistance due to progesterone, can result in the woman feeling faint or fainting, resolved quickly by repositioning the woman on her side or in a lateral position.
- An increase in blood volume through haemodilution (increasing by 45%) occurs together with a small increase in the numbers of red blood cells. The disproportionate increase in plasma volume relative to the increase in red cell mass can lead to a 'physiological' anaemia in the mother from around 27 weeks gestation. Due to the increase in blood volume, a pregnant woman is able to tolerate greater blood loss before showing signs of hypovolaemia. This compensation is at the expense of shunting blood away from the uterus and placenta, and therefore the fetus.
- Overall increase in blood volume results in a pregnant woman being able to tolerate greater blood loss before showing signs of hypovolaemia.

Respiratory system:
- An increase in breathing rate and effort and decrease in vital capacity, as the gravid uterus enlarges and the diaphragm becomes splinted.
- Some shortness of breath is common during pregnancy, but early consideration should be given to the need for increased oxygen requirements.
- Oedema of the larynx may compromise airway management and a collapsed pregnant woman requires the airway to be managed and secured as soon as possible.

Gastrointestinal system:
● Nausea and vomiting can occur around 4–8 weeks gestation and continue until around 14–16 weeks. Some severe cases may continue for a longer period of time and can result in rapid dehydration (hyperemesis gravidarum) requiring hospital assessment/admission. Relaxation of the cardiac sphincter makes regurgitation of the stomach contents more likely.
● An increase in the acidity of the stomach contents, due to a delay in gastric emptying, caused by progesterone-like effects of the placental hormones.

Structured Assessment

Every woman will require an immediate visual inspection by the attending responder. The first step involves the primary survey (Table 2.1), which aims to identify any life-threatening

	Are there any immediately life-threatening problems? Is it safe to approach the woman?
Airway	Is the woman able to talk? (Yes = airway open.)
	Is the woman making unusual sounds? (Gurgling = fluid in the airway.)
	Is wiping or suction required? (Snoring = tongue/swelling/vomit/foreign body obstruction.)
	If the woman is unresponsive, open the airway and look in – wipe away or suction fluids, manually remove solid obstructions.

Table 2.1 Primary survey

Chapter 2

	Are there any immediately life-threatening problems? Is it safe to approach the woman?
Breathing	What is the respiratory rate and effort? (Are accessory muscles being used?)
	Obtain oxygen saturations (if probe available).
	Auscultate for added sounds if trained to do so. (Wheeze = bronchospasm; coarse sounds = pulmonary oedema.)
	Assess for the presence of cyanosis.
Circulation	Feel radial pulse rate and volume.
	Assess skin colour and temperature (to touch). (Pallor, or cold or damp skin.)
	Record blood pressure if equipped.
	Visually inspect the abdominal area and gently palpate for evidence of internal bleeding (indicated by tenderness, guarding or firm 'woody' uterus).
Massive haemorrhage	Is there a significant volume of blood visible?
	Are the clothes soaked or floor covered with blood?

Table 2.1 (*continued*)

	Are there any immediately life-threatening problems? Is it safe to approach the woman?
Disability	Perform an **AVPU** assessment: • Is she **A**lert? • Only responding to **V**oice? • Only responding to **P**ain? • **U**nresponsive? Observe the woman's posture (normal, convulsing (state whether focal or generalised), abnormal flexion, abnormal extension). Inspect pupil size and reaction (PEaRL – pupils equal and reacting to light). Consider blood glucose measurement.
Exposure/ **E**nvironment/ **E**valuate	Ask the woman's consent to visually inspect the vaginal opening: • Is there any evidence of bleeding? • Can you see a presenting part of the baby? • Is there a prolapsed loop of cord? • Have the waters broken (and if so, is the amniotic fluid clear, blood-stained, meconium-stained or malodorous)? • Does the perineum bulge with each contraction? • If the baby has been born, is there a significant perineal tear? Can you see any part of the uterus?

Table 2.1 (*continued*)

Chapter 2

	Are there any immediately life-threatening problems? Is it safe to approach the woman?
	Assess the environment: • Are the woman and/or baby at risk of hypothermia? • Are the surroundings as clean as you can make them if the birth is imminent? • Are there other children present (this may indicate a previous pregnancy with live birth)? Evaluate how time critical the woman's condition is. If it is time critical, decide immediately whether you need to transport the woman urgently to the nearest hospital with an obstetric facility. If the birth is imminent, remember to call for help. This may include midwifery or medical assistance if available locally.
Fundus/**F**etus	Make a quick assessment of fundal height: a fundus at the level of the umbilicus equates to a gestation of approximately 22 weeks, see Figure 2.1. By definition, if fundal height is below the umbilicus, this suggests that if the fetus is delivered, it is unlikely to survive. Is the woman experiencing regular, painful contractions? Ask the woman when she last felt the baby move/kick, was this a normal pattern for her baby?

Table 2.1   (*continued*)

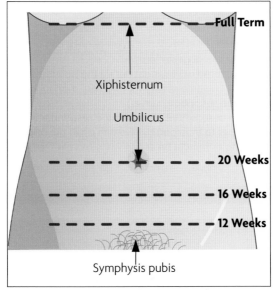

Xiphisternum

Umbilicus

Full Term

20 Weeks

16 Weeks

12 Weeks

Symphysis pubis

Figure 2.1   Fundal height.

problems, enable management to commence as rapidly as possible and to reach an early decision regarding whether to take the woman to the nearest health facility or await the impending birth.

If any critical problems are identified during the primary survey, the secondary survey should only be undertaken when any **ABCDEF** problems have been addressed and transportation to an appropriate facility has commenced (if this is possible). In many cases where critical problems are identified, it will not be possible or appropriate to undertake a secondary survey in the pre-hospital phase of care.

Key Points for Assessment of the Pregnant Woman

- Maternal changes in response to pregnancy can occur as early as 4–6 weeks of gestation.
- Using a structured assessment during the primary survey will ensure that any time critical features are managed prior to moving on to the secondary survey.
- A structured assessment will guide the responder in deciding whether to transport the woman on to the appropriate obstetric facility or remain on scene while the birth takes place.

Chapter 3
Bleeding in Pregnancy

Bleeding in pregnancy is broadly divided into two timeframes: bleeding that occurs in the early part of pregnancy (less than 24 weeks), such as miscarriage or ectopic pregnancy, and that occurring in the late second and third trimesters of pregnancy (after 24 weeks), such as placenta praevia or placental abruption. See Figure 3.1 for examples of blood volumes in different sanitary towels.

Any bleeding from the genital tract during pregnancy is of concern and in early pregnancy may indicate miscarriage or an

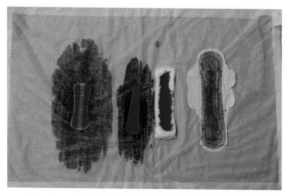

Figure 3.1   *Four sanitary towels, each soaked with 50 ml blood.*

ectopic pregnancy. This more commonly occurs in the first three months (weeks 1–12) but can also occur in the second trimester.

Haemorrhage may:
- present with evident vaginal loss of blood (e.g. miscarriage and placenta praevia); or
- occur mainly (or completely) within the abdomen or uterus. This presents with little or no external loss, but pain and signs of hypovolaemic shock (e.g. ruptured ectopic pregnancy and placental abruption).

Alternatively, a pregnant woman may appear well even with a large amount of concealed blood loss. Increase in maternal heart rate (tachycardia) may not appear until 30% or more of the circulating volume has been depleted.

Bleeding in Early Pregnancy: Less than 24 Weeks

Miscarriage is most common in the first 12 weeks of gestation (commonly 6–14 weeks). The woman will often be anxious as to what is happening and can be very concerned as to the health and well-being of her unborn baby.

Problems associated with miscarriage occur when some of the early fetal or placental tissues (known as 'products of conception') are partly passed through the cervix and may become trapped, leading to continuing blood loss. If shock ensues, it is often out of proportion to the amount of blood loss (i.e. there is an added vagal (nerve) stimulation from tissue trapped in the cervix). In all women of childbearing age, have a high index of suspicion for ectopic pregnancy or ectopic rupture if they have the symptoms outlined below.

Risk factors:
- Previous history of miscarriage.
- Previously identified potential miscarriage at scan.

- Smoking.
- Obesity.

Symptoms:
- Bleeding: light or heavy, often with clots and/or 'jelly-like' tissue.
- Pain: central, crampy, suprapubic or backache.
- Signs of pregnancy may be subsiding, e.g. nausea or breast tenderness.
- Significant symptoms (including hypotension) without obvious external blood loss may indicate 'cervical shock' due to miscarriage tissue retained in the cervix. Symptomatic slow maternal heart rate (bradycardia) may arise due to vagal stimulation.
- Usually presents at around 6–8 weeks gestation, so usually only one period has been missed.

Symptoms characteristic of a ruptured ectopic pregnancy:
- Acute lower abdominal pain.
- Slight bleeding or brownish vaginal discharge.
- Signs of blood loss within the abdomen with tachycardia and skin coolness.

Other suspicious symptoms and risk factors:
- Unexplained fainting.
- Shoulder-tip pain.
- Unusual bowel symptoms.
- Intra-uterine contraceptive device fitted.
- Previous ectopic pregnancy.
- Previous tubal surgery.
- Sterilisation or reversal of sterilisation.
- Endometriosis.
- Pelvic inflammatory disease.
- Subfertility (delay in conceiving).

Bleeding in Late Pregnancy: More than 24 Weeks

Antepartum or peripartum haemorrhage (> 24 weeks) may indicate placenta praevia or placental abruption.

Placenta praevia

Occurs in 1 in 200 pregnancies and usually presents at 24–32 weeks with small episodes of painless bleeding. The placenta develops low down in the uterus and partially or completely covers the internal opening of the cervical canal, the internal cervical os, see Figure 3.2. With the development and growth of the uterus, bleeding is inevitable. This can lead to severe haemorrhage during the pregnancy (i.e. painless bleeding) or when labour begins.

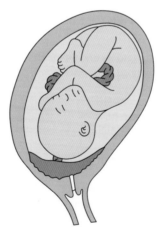

Figure 3.2   Placenta praevia.

Placental abruption

Any vaginal bleeding in late pregnancy (after 24 weeks) or during labour which is accompanied by severe/sudden continuous abdominal/back pain, or with signs of shock, may be due to placental abruption, see Figure 3.3. Bleeding occurs between the placenta and the wall of the uterus, detaching an area of the placenta from the uterine wall. Blood may either be contained in a pouch formed by the placental-uterine separation or bleed freely. Hence, an abruption can result in either evident visible blood loss (revealed) or non-visible loss (concealed). It can be associated with severe pregnancy-induced hypertension (PIH) and trauma. Placental abruption causes continuous severe/sudden abdominal/back pain and tightening of the uterus and/or signs of hypovolaemic shock, and puts the unborn baby at immediate risk. There

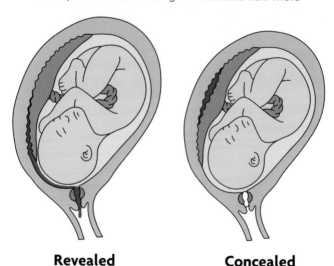

Revealed   **Concealed**

Figure 3.3   *Placental abruption: revealed and concealed.*

may be some external blood loss, but more commonly the haemorrhage is **concealed** behind the placenta. Where there is a combination of **revealed** (external) blood loss and concealed haemorrhage, this can be particularly dangerous, as it can lead to an underestimation of the amount of total blood lost. The woman's abdomen will be tender when felt and the uterus will feel rigid or 'woody' with no signs of relaxation.

Because the true amount of bleeding is concealed, placental abruption is also associated with disseminated intravascular coagulation (DIC), which can worsen the tendency to bleed. Placental abruption can be immediately life-threatening to both the woman and the unborn baby.

Key Points for Bleeding in Pregnancy

- Haemorrhage during pregnancy is broadly divided into two categories, occurring in early and late pregnancy.
- Haemorrhage may be revealed (evident vaginal blood loss) or concealed (little or no obvious loss).
- Pregnant women may appear well even when a large amount of blood has been lost; tachycardia may not appear until 30% of circulating volume has been depleted, and symptoms of hypovolaemic shock occur very late, by which stage the woman is critical.

Chapter 4

Emergency Birth

The best clinical management for a woman who presents in established labour is transportation to the nearest appropriate facility without delay. This will usually be the nearest maternity or obstetric unit, but in certain circumstances may involve transfer to the nearest ED.

Where there is access to specialist health professionals, such as midwives or an obstetrician in an antenatal clinic, their assistance should be sought. If the birth is not immediately imminent, arranging transport for the woman to the nearest facility, with appropriately trained staff, is the priority of care.

When attending a pregnant woman, where birth is not imminent and there are no complications, it may be appropriate to contact the midwife or physician in the booked maternity unit for advice regarding the transport arrangements. This may involve the woman making her own way to her planned place of birth, if there are no immediate time critical features.

The most important feature of attending a pregnant woman is to complete a rapid assessment, as detailed in Chapter 2, to ascertain whether birth is imminent.

Additional assessment should include the following:
● Establish the gestation of the pregnancy and whether, if born, the baby will be premature.

- Ask the woman if she has received maternity care and if she has electronic or hand-held maternity records.
- Identify any risk factors or complications early on.
- Assess for:
  o a blood-stained 'show' or mucous plug lost from the cervix;
  o ruptured amniotic fluid ('waters broken'), noting colour, i.e. blood-stained or green indicating meconium;
  o contractions and their frequency; and/or
  o bleeding.
- If none of the above are present, contact the local maternity care provider for advice regarding ongoing management.
- If indicated, and with the consent of the woman, undertake a visual inspection of the vaginal opening if there are regular contractions (1–2-minute intervals) and an urge to push or bear down.

If the birth is imminent, you will need to prepare the following:
- Ensure the privacy of the environment, and instruct those around you to safeguard the dignity of the woman.
- Ensure the environment is as warm as possible, reducing drafts where possible (the ideal room temperature is around 25° Celsius).
- Cover the area where the birth is about to take place, using a clean towel or a sheet.
- Gather clean, soft items, either towels or sheets, that can be pre-warmed (these can be placed inside the clothing of a person if the birth is outside) and used to dry the baby immediately following the birth.
- If you have a prepared 'maternity response' pack, open accordingly and lay out.

Normal Mechanism of Labour

The fetus is an active part of the normal labour process, becoming more flexed during the birth. With increasing contractions the fetus will descend further in the pelvis. As the newborn head becomes visible under the pubic arch, the head is described as 'crowning'. The extension of the fetal head results in the birth of the baby's face and chin. As the newborn head realigns itself in relation to its shoulders (restitution), the head appears to rotate with the baby toward the mother's inner thigh. As the shoulders navigate the pelvis, they rotate into the wide diameter of the pelvis at its outlet, and further rotation of the newborn head can be seen. The body will birth with either the anterior or the posterior shoulder presenting and it may be necessary to support the birth of the baby as this takes place.

During a normal birth:
- Support the woman in a position in which she is comfortable, this should not be on her back if this is not her preference. Women naturally adopt a range of positions including on all-fours, on their side, or kneeling.
- Provide support and reassurance while maintaining privacy and dignity.
- Encourage the mother to breathe slowly and work together; make eye contact.
- Provide pain relief if the woman chooses and this is available.
- Allow the baby's head to be born slowly, encourage the woman to concentrate on breathing slowly during the birth of the head and panting if necessary.
- Some responders may consider applying gentle pressure to the top of the baby's head as it advances through the vagina to prevent very rapid birth. Gentle pressure may also assist in keeping the newborn head flexed, possibly reducing trauma to the perineum. Once the head is born, the birth of the baby is normally complete in the next two contractions or up to 2 minutes.

- Avoid touching the umbilical cord during the birth, it may be obvious around the baby's neck, but the baby can be born without it being interrupted or touched. Never suction the baby's mouth or nose when the head has just birthed, as this could stimulate the baby and is of no proven benefit at this time.
- As the baby is born, pass to the mother, preferably onto her abdomen.
- Wipe any obvious collections of mucous from the baby's mouth and nose.
- Thoroughly dry the baby using the warm towel, placing the baby's skin directly next to the mother's once the baby is completely dry.
- Once the baby is next to the maternal skin, wrap the second towel around the mother and the baby to protect from draught, ensuring the baby's head is covered but not the face (see Figure 4.1).
- Assess the baby while next to the maternal skin.

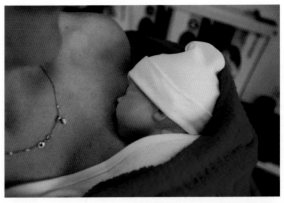

Figure 4.1 *Newborn baby with head covered, skin-to-skin with mother.*

● All babies are at risk of low body temperature (hypothermia) but those born prematurely lose heat faster than those born after 37 weeks gestation.

After the birth:

● Keep the baby with its mother in a position where the mother can breastfeed if she wants to (breastfeeding will also encourage birth of the placenta).

● Wait until the umbilical cord has stopped pulsating, and if your maternity response kit allows, apply two cord clamps securely 3 cm apart and 15 cm from the newborn umbilicus. The cord can then be cut between the two clamps (Figure 4.2). (Caution: ensure the baby's fingers and genitals are clear of the scissors.)

● Reassure the mother, and offer congratulations if appropriate; it is important to remember that while the birth was unplanned at the location, it remains a very important celebration.

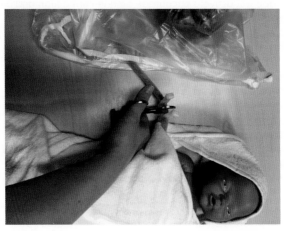

Figure 4.2   *Positioning of clamps on the umbilical cord.*

- Do not await the birth of the placenta if the local service does not provide for a midwife or physician to attend the location.
- The priority is to ensure that assessment of the mother and the baby takes places as soon as possible by the most appropriate professional, i.e. a midwife, obstetrician, obstetric nurse or physician. The attending professional will be determined by the local healthcare system.
- If the birth has occurred while transferring the mother to hospital, ensure the receiving obstetric or medical facility is contacted to inform them that both mother and baby/babies will be arriving together where appropriate.
- The mother may report further contractions prior to expulsion of the placenta, assist further by encouraging her to adopt a squatting or upright position and catch the placenta into a bag or a bowl.
- Encourage the mother to empty her bladder to facilitate uterine contraction and control further bleeding. Breastfeeding the baby will actively encourage uterine contraction and birth of the placenta.
- Do not pull the umbilical cord during birth of the placenta as this could rupture the cord, making birth of the placenta difficult, and cause excessive bleeding or inversion of the uterus.
- Once the placenta is born keep it in a bowl or plastic bag, together with any blood and membranes, ready for inspection by a midwife or respective obstetric clinician.
- Note that if the placenta has not been born within 20 minutes of birth, there is an increased risk of haemorrhage. If it is within the skillset of the responder, an intravenous cannula is indicated and the woman may require intravenous fluid and further intervention (oxytocic's).
- If bleeding continues after birth of the placenta, palpate the mother's abdomen and feel for the top of the uterus (fundus), usually at the level of the umbilicus, and massage firmly with

a cupped hand in a circular motion, known as 'rubbing up a contraction' or fundal massage.

- The fundus will become firm as massage is applied and this may be quite uncomfortable, so painkillers should be offered if available.
- Be aware that the uterus may relax again and bleeding recommence. 'Rubbing up a contraction' may need to be repeated.
- In preparation for transportation, provide a sanitary towel (if available) and encourage the woman to put on her underwear, keeping the mother and baby warm together while waiting for the appropriate assessment by the midwife or physician.

Key Points for Emergency Birth

- If the woman is experiencing contractions at 1–2-minute intervals, has an urge to bear down or push, complete a visual inspection of the vaginal opening to confirm the birth is imminent.
- Allow the birth of the baby's head to take place slowly, to minimise the likelihood of perineal trauma.
- Ensure the baby is thoroughly dried and given skin-to-skin contact with the mother as soon as possible to help maintain newborn temperature and facilitate the birth of the placenta.

Chapter 5
Pre-term Birth

Prematurity is defined as less than 37 completed weeks of pregnancy. Premature babies are more likely to need assistance with breathing and maintaining their own temperature.

At less than 32 weeks of gestation, spontaneous breathing will be inadequate, and these babies are likely to be deficient in surfactant (surfactant reduces alveolar surface tension and keeps the lung alveoli open during expiration), necessitating surfactant replacement and/or ventilatory support, and immediate transfer to the nearest obstetric unit or ED.

In babies less than 32 weeks gestation, there is an increased risk of intracranial bleeding (bleeding occurring within the brain).

Other complications of prematurity include hypothermia, hypoglycaemia and a higher risk of infection.

Improving neonatal intensive care has seen better outcomes for babies born pre-term (especially in babies born after 28 weeks gestation). However, the EPICure2 study, following up on babies born in the UK at the limits of viability before 26 weeks gestation, showed high mortality and morbidity. Overall survival was only 39% and survivors commonly have severe disabilities. Hypothermia was one of the factors associated with death. Ensure the newborn baby is dried as detailed earlier and has skin-to-skin contact with the mother. Neonatal wraps or foil cribs can be used if available in the responder's maternity kit.

Birth at Less Than 24 Weeks Gestation

Responders may attend births at extremes of prematurity and viability. The guidance regarding newborn resuscitation in the pre-hospital phase of care is less well defined than in an obstetric unit, where access to neonatal expertise can enable a plan to be discussed with the woman based upon the clinical assessment of the pregnancy to date. Different health systems may have defined guidance for pre-hospital clinicians at the extremes of gestation and as such the responder should familiarise themselves with local policies and procedures. The following guidance acts to enable responders working in the pre-hospital setting to be supported when faced with a baby born prematurely between 20 and 24 weeks gestation.

● When attending a birth at 20–24 weeks OR the gestation is unknown, and there are signs of life, the recommendations are:

○ Dry the baby with one towel and then wrap in a new warm towel or blanket. Ensure the head is covered with a small baby hat if available.

○ Maintain ventilations using the smallest paediatric mask available.

○ Provide effective ventilations with the baby lying flat, assess heart rate and do not expect the chest to move at this gestation. If ventilations are effective the heart rate will remain stable or improve.

○ Where neonatal wraps or cribs are available these should be used to minimise heat loss.

○ Place a pre-arrival information phone call stating the gestation of the baby if known, and whether the mother is travelling with the baby.

o Convey to the nearest appropriate obstetric or hospital facility, requesting the neonatal team (the needs of the pre-term baby are a priority at this gestation until a specialised assessment is made of the baby and its chances of survival).

● Where there are signs of life, ventilations should be continued until the neonatal team can assess the gestation and weight of the baby. The team will then consider the ongoing management in the best interests of the baby and the family.

● A responder should not discontinue resuscitative attempts; this decision sits within the expertise of the neonatologist.

● A baby born at less than 20 weeks gestation can be either given to the mother to hold, or if the mother prefers not to hold the baby, placed in a soft item, and given to the clinician at the nearest appropriate facility depending upon local health service configuration (this may be an early pregnancy, gynaecology or maternity service).

● If the birth has taken place en route to hospital, both mother and baby should be taken to the nearest appropriate facility.

● At 20–37 weeks gestation, transfer the woman to the nearest obstetric unit or ED with an obstetric unit dependent on local policy, as the baby will require specialist assessment by the neonatal team once born.

● Keeping the baby warm is a priority in the pre-term newborn.

● In some circumstances, it may be necessary to convey the baby separately from the mother, dependent upon the clinical condition of either newborn or mother. In this instance, mother and baby should be conveyed to the same location where possible.

● A pre-arrival information call should be placed to the facility informing them of the gestation of the newborn baby where known (including whether the mother is accompanying the newborn baby in the vehicle).

Key Points for Pre-term Birth

- Babies born at less than 37 weeks are more likely to require assistance with their breathing and maintaining their body temperature.
- It may be necessary to convey the baby separately from the mother, dependent upon the clinical condition of either the newborn or the mother.
- A pre-arrival information call should include the gestation of the baby at birth, and whether the mother is accompanying the baby in the same vehicle.

Chapter 6

Umbilical Cord Prolapse

A prolapsed umbilical cord is a **time critical emergency** for the unborn baby. The descent of the umbilical cord, through the uterine cervix and into the vagina may be recognised by the woman after her 'waters' have broken. She may report the sensation of 'something' in the vagina, or an obvious length of the umbilical cord hanging down when she goes to the toilet.

While the umbilical cord remains prolapsed, the presenting part of the unborn baby (whether head or bottom) can cause compression upon the cord, and subsequently interfere with adequate oxygenation of the unborn baby until the pressure is relieved.

Upon identification of a prolapsed umbilical cord, the priorities are to:
- facilitate maternal positioning to relieve the pressure of the fetal presenting part off the umbilical cord. Instruct the woman to adopt a knee to chest position on the floor with her buttocks high in the air (Figure 6.1);
- avoid handling the umbilical cord to reduce the chances of the blood vessels within the cord becoming constricted. Use a dry pad or sanitary towel and gently place the cord back into the woman's vagina (the vagina is warm and moist, which will avoid the cord becoming cold and dry, causing vasoconstriction of the cord);
- walk the woman quickly to the waiting ambulance, avoid any upright seated positions, including the use of the carry

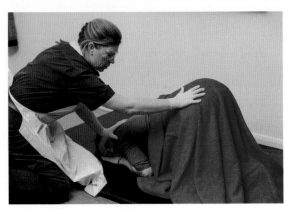

Figure 6.1 *Knee chest position.*

chair, that will cause gravity to direct the pressure of the fetal presenting part onto the umbilical cord; and

• transfer the woman to the nearest obstetric or medical facility where the birth can be expedited (this will usually be by caesarean section, unless birth is imminent upon arrival).

In certain areas, a trained clinician may be available to offer the emergency intervention of 'bladder filling'. This involves a midwife or physician passing a catheter into the maternal bladder, filling it with a volume of fluid, and then clamping the catheter to ensure the bladder cannot empty. While this can be uncomfortable for the woman, filling the bladder lifts the presenting part of the unborn baby off the umbilical cord. This intervention can also inhibit uterine contractions if the woman is in labour at the time of the cord prolapse. Bladder filling can offer valuable time to relieve pressure from the umbilical cord, particularly where access to a medical facility is likely to include a lengthy journey. While this intervention may not

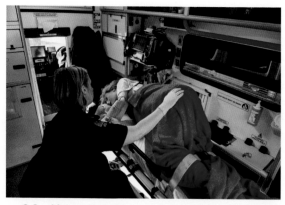

Figure 6.2   Maternal positioning during transport to hospital.

be within the scope of a responder, access to a pre-hospital medical team may afford this intervention to be undertaken.

Transfer of the woman in a vehicle should involve her lying on her side, with a cushion to elevate her lowest hip (encourage the presenting part of the unborn baby to descend out of the pelvis and thus relieve pressure on the cord), as demonstrated in Figure 6.2. This is preferably in a lateral position facing her accompanying clinician who can provide ongoing reassurance.

A pre-arrival information call should include the obstetric emergency 'cord prolapse'. This aids the receiving clinicians to mobilise the necessary team ready for arrival of the woman.

Key Points for Umbilical Cord Prolapse

- If waiting for transportation, position the woman in the 'knee chest' position to relieve pressure on the umbilical cord. During transfer the woman should adopt a lateral position with her lower hip elevated.

• 'Bladder filling' can be considered if within the scope of the responder and journey times to the appropriate facility are lengthy.

• A pre-alert information call should include the obstetric emergency of '**cord prolapse**'.

Chapter 7
Shoulder Dystocia

The term 'shoulder dystocia' is used to describe the arrest of spontaneous birth. Once the newborn head is delivered, the anterior shoulder of the baby becomes impacted against the maternal symphysis pubis and requires early recognition and timely interventions, to expedite birth and avoid any potential sequelae to the baby.

Shoulder dystocia is a **time critical** emergency and requires a systematic approach to enable the birth of the baby. Consider an early request for a midwife and a pre-hospital team where available.

The objectives of interventions used to facilitate the birth are to:
● enhance the pelvic diameters by changing the maternal position and using the McRoberts position. See Figure 7.1;
● reduce the bi-sacromial diameters (fetal shoulders) to aid birth by the use of suprapubic pressure. See Figure 7.2;
● rotate the fetal shoulders into the oblique diameter of the pelvis to aid birth. This can be achieved with the use of suprapubic pressure.

Following the birth of the newborn head, the shoulders rotate into the anterior–posterior position within the maternal pelvis and birth normally takes place with the next two uterine contractions.

If any the following occur, an attempt must be made to deliver the shoulders:
● The shoulders are not born within two contractions following the birth of the head.
● There is difficulty with birth of the face and chin.
● The head remains tightly applied to the vulva or retracts ('turtle-neck' sign).
● There is a failure of the head to fully rotate to face towards the woman's inner thigh once born.

Call for help if you are on your own, as you will need additional assistance.

Undertake the McRoberts manoeuvre, which alters the angle of the pelvis (Figures 7.1 and 7.2).
1. Ask the woman to lie flat and bring her bottom to the end of the bed.
2. Bring the woman's knees up on to her abdomen (the legs will naturally abduct due to the pregnant uterus).

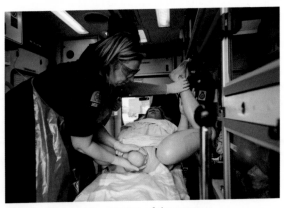

Figure 7.1 *McRoberts position of the woman.*

If available, use a helper (this can be the partner or another person) to support each leg or ask the woman to hold them.

3. Ask the woman to push with the next contraction. This may release the shoulders and enable the birth to proceed.

4. If the shoulders do not release during the contraction, the responder should attempt to deliver the baby's shoulders with gentle 'axial' traction applied to the baby's head (this is outward traction keeping the baby's head in line with its own spine, and is angled just below horizontal); the woman is encouraged to push. AVOID pulling the baby's head downwards or laterally towards the floor and avoid twisting the baby's neck at any time (this can damage the brachial plexus nerves).

5. If the baby remains undelivered after **30 seconds**, move on to applying suprapubic pressure while the woman remains in the McRoberts position.

Use of suprapubic pressure (Figure 7.2):

- Identify where the fetal back is facing.

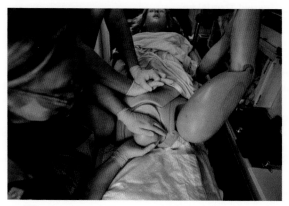

Figure 7.2   *Applying suprapubic pressure.*

- Ask your helper to:
  ○ stand on the maternal side where the baby's back is (if the baby's back is facing left, stand on the woman's left, or vice versa);
  ○ place their hands in a CPR-style grip with the heel of the hand two finger breaths above the maternal symphysis pubic (pubic bone);
  ○ apply moderate pressure in a downwards and lateral direction **continuously** for **30 seconds**; and
  ○ encourage the woman to push to attempt gentle axial traction to deliver the baby.
- If the shoulders DO NOT release:
  ○ attempt **intermittent** suprapubic pressure for a further **30 seconds**;
  ○ ask the helper to apply intermittent pressure on the shoulder by rocking gently backwards and forwards;
  ○ encourage the woman to push or attempt gentle axial traction to deliver the baby;
  ○ if unsuccessful, change the woman's position to 'all fours'.

'All Fours' Position

(For the lone attending responder this is an ideal first position to use as it provides a very effective McRoberts manoeuvre.)

- Position the woman on her hands and knees with her hips well flexed (any movement of the pelvis may help release the shoulders).
- Encourage the woman to push to release shoulders or apply gentle axial traction to release the shoulder nearest to the maternal back first.
- If unsuccessful, transfer the woman to the transport vehicle; she may be walked as this may also encourage the birth. Responders should be prepared to anticipate the birth during transfer and/or conveyance.

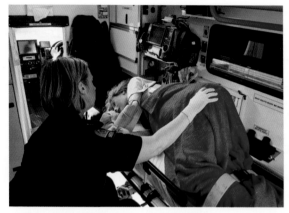

Figure 7.3   *Position of woman during transfer.*

- Convey the woman to the nearest obstetric or medical unit positioned in a lateral position using a pillow to separate the woman's legs and avoid pressure on the baby's head (Figure 7.3). Offer Entonox to provide analgesia if required.
- Place a pre-arrival information call stating the obstetric emergency of '**shoulder dystocia**'. It may be necessary to request staff meet at a suitable entrance to avoid any delays due to accessing buildings or lifts.

The use of internal manoeuvres by responders:

- Where McRoberts manoeuvre, suprapubic pressure and all fours position have been attempted to expedite the birth, the use of specific internal manoeuvres may be appropriate, if a responder has received additional training to undertake them.
- In a pre-hospital setting where a lone attending responder is first on scene, the use of the all fours position may facilitate the removal of the posterior arm, notably when awaiting an ambulance or other transport to arrive at the scene.

Key Points for Shoulder Dystocia

- Shoulder dystocia is a time critical emergency and requires a systematic approach to enable the timely birth of the baby by the use of:

    1. McRoberts position;
    2. suprapubic pressure;
    3. all fours position;
    4. internal manoeuvres where within the scope of the responder.

- Each intervention should be attempted for up to 30 seconds.

- A pre-arrival information call should include the obstetric emergency '**shoulder dystocia**'.

Chapter 8

Breech Birth

Vaginal breech birth is where the feet or buttocks of the baby present first rather than the baby's head. Cord prolapse is more common with a breech presentation.

Vaginal breech birth – if birth is **NOT** in progress:
- Recognise breech presentation (may be documented in the woman's antenatal notes, thick meconium may be seen at vaginal opening, fetal buttocks or feet may be visible at vaginal opening).
- Transfer woman to the nearest obstetric or medical facility without delay.
- Constantly re-assess en route and take appropriate action if the circumstances change.

Vaginal breech birth – if birth **IS** in progress:
- Request a midwife and the pre-hospital team (if available locally) and additional help. Consider an early request for a midwife and a pre-hospital team.
- Prepare for newborn resuscitation.
- Encourage the woman to adopt a suitable position for gravity to help the birth of the baby, e.g. resting on the edge of the bed or the edge of a sofa or the 'all fours' position.
- The optimal position for the breech birth is for the baby's back to remain uppermost to the maternal abdomen OR 'baby's tum towards Mum's bum'. See Figure 8.1 for an illustration of a breech birth position.

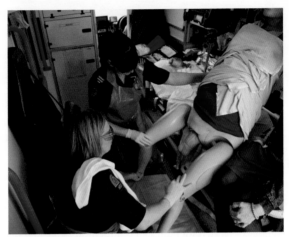

Figure 8.1 *Breech birth with woman seated on edge of the trolley bed (note position of the fetal back is uppermost to the maternal abdomen).*

- Allow the breech to descend spontaneously with maternal pushing, and maintain a 'hands off' approach to the birth. (It is not necessary to touch the baby or handle the umbilical cord during the birth.)
- The baby's legs and arms will spontaneously birth and do not require assistance.
- Only assist to ensure the baby's back remains uppermost to the maternal abdomen – 'baby's tum towards Mum's bum'.
- If the baby's back rotates away from the woman's abdomen, gently handle the baby over the hips (bony pelvis) and gently rotate the baby's back to face towards the maternal abdomen.
- If the woman is in a semi-recumbent position, once the baby's body is born to the nape of the neck, allow the birth of the head to take place slowly. The head can be supported by

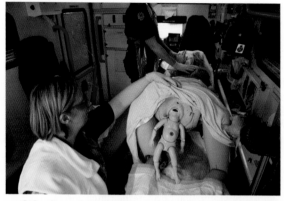

Figure 8.2   Breech birth in the 'all fours' position (note the fetal back towards the maternal abdomen).

placing the body of the baby on the responder's forearm and gently lifting the baby to facilitate the birth of the baby's head.
• If the woman is in the 'all fours' position (Figure 8.2), as the head is born, the baby can be born into the responder's hands and passed through the mother's legs for her to hold.
• Once the birth is complete, if the baby does not require any resuscitation, management of the baby and the umbilical cord should be as per normal birth guidelines and the cord should be left to stop pulsating.
• Breech babies are more likely to be covered in meconium and may require resuscitation.

If delays occur during the birth:
• Legs: If the legs delay birth of the body, apply gentle pressure to the back of the baby's knee (popliteal fossa), gently allow the leg to naturally abduct outward enabling birth of each individual leg.

- Arms: If the arms are extended, gently rotate the baby's pelvis 90° and aid delivery of the first (uppermost) arm, then rotate the baby in the opposite direction 180° and release the other arm.
- If the head does not deliver in the semi-recumbent position (with the baby's body supported on your forearm), apply pressure to the back of the baby's head with the fingers of your other hand, to aid flexion while the head delivers.
- Where responders have received appropriate training in management of breech birth, additional manoeuvres can be undertaken as detailed above for management of the legs, arms and head where delay in birth is identified.
- Where the responder has not received appropriate training, the nearest obstetric unit or obstetric physician may be contacted to provide guidance on the ongoing management.
- Any presenting body part other than the head, buttocks or feet (e.g. one foot or hand/arm):
  - Transfer the woman immediately to the nearest obstetric or medical facility and provide a pre-arrival information call reporting the obstetric emergency of '**foot/arm presentation**'.
  - It may be necessary to request staff to meet you at an agreed location to ensure rapid assessment and management of the woman.

Key Points for Breech Birth

- The optimal position for the breech birth is for the baby's back to remain uppermost to the maternal abdomen OR 'baby's tum towards Mum's bum'.
- Babies born in the breech position are more likely to be covered in meconium and may require resuscitation.
- Allow the breech to descend spontaneously with maternal pushing and maintain a 'hands off' approach to the birth.

Chapter 9

Post-partum Haemorrhage

Post-partum haemorrhage (PPH) is the most common cause of severe haemorrhage immediately after birth due to uterine atony (poor contraction of the uterus). There are four common reasons for primary post-partum haemorrhage as detailed in Table 9.1.

Primary PPH can occur within the first 24 hours after birth and is defined as a blood loss of 500 ml or more within this timeframe. Secondary PPH can occur from 24 hours up to 3 months after birth (Figure 9.1).

	Specific cause	Relative frequency
Tone	Atonic uterus	70%
Trauma	Cervical, vaginal, perineal lacerations	20%
	Pelvic haematoma	
	Inverted uterus	
	Uterine rupture	
Tissue	Retained tissue	10%
	Invasive placenta	
Thrombin	Coagulopathies	1%

Table 9.1 The 4 "T's" of primary post-partum haemorrhage

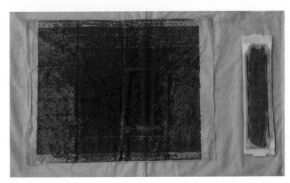

Figure 9.1   *Maternity pad with 500 ml blood and sanitary pad with 50 ml blood.*

After birth the uterus should contract to control haemorrhage, and the responder can feel the uterus harden by palpating the mother's abdomen. The uterus can often be described as well contracted if it feels like the 'hardness' of a cricket ball or a firm piece of fruit.

If the uterus is found to be soft, or flaccid, it is then described as 'atonic' and the management of this should as follows.

If the placenta **has delivered**:
● Palpate the maternal abdomen and feel for the top of the uterus (fundus), usually at the level of the maternal umbilicus, and massage firmly with a cupped hand in a circular motion (known as 'rubbing up a contraction' or uterine massage):
    1. The responder cups their hand against the uterus at the level of the symphysis pubis to support the uterus.
    2. The other hand is cupped and actively massages the uterus toward the other hand.
● The top of the uterus should become firm as massage is applied, see Figure 9.2. It can be very uncomfortable for the

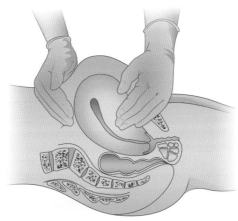

Figure 9.2   Uterine massage.

mother and may be necessary to offer pain relief. In the UK the most common analgesia is Entonox.
● If within the scope of the role of the responder, the administration of an 'uterotonic' (a drug that will aid uterine contraction, e.g. Syntometrine or misoprostol) can be considered.
● Empty the bladder by encouraging the woman to sit on a bed pan, where available, rather than the toilet.
● If within the scope of the role of the responder, gaining intravenous access early is critical.
● Convey to the nearest obstetric or medical facility.

If the placenta **has not delivered**:
● In the presence of haemorrhage, do not massage the top of the uterus (fundus) when the placenta is undelivered. This may provoke partial separation of the placenta and cause further

Chapter 9

haemorrhage. (In the event of life-threatening haemorrhage, massaging the uterus may be necessary.)

● If within the scope of the responder, consider administration of a 'uterotonic' drug. In the UK, the most common drug used is Syntometrine (an intramuscular injection containing oxytocin and ergometrine).

● Other drugs may be indicated, and local health systems will need to have an agreed protocol to which drug regimen is recommended.

● If within the scope of the role of the responder, gaining intravenous access early is critical.

● If the placenta delivers while transporting the woman to hospital, be prepared to undertake uterine massage, 'rubbing up a contraction', if the woman continues to bleed.

● Convey to the nearest obstetric or medical facility, providing a pre-arrival information call detailing '**post-partum haemorrhage**'.

● If the mother continues to bleed, despite the uterus being well contracted, visually inspect the vaginal opening to assess for any obvious perineal trauma. If present, apply direct manual pressure using a gauze or maternity pad.

Key Points for Post-partum Haemorrhage

● After birth the uterus should contract to control haemorrhage.

● If the uterus is found to be soft or flaccid, palpate the maternal abdomen, feel for the top of the uterus and perform uterine massage.

● Convey to the nearest obstetric or medical facility providing a pre-arrival information call detailing '**post-partum haemorrhage**'.

Chapter 10

Convulsions During Pregnancy or After Birth

Eclampsia is generalised tonic/clonic convulsions and visually identical to an epileptic convulsion. Many women presenting with eclampsia will have had pre-existing pre-eclampsia (of a mild, moderate or severe degree), but some cases of eclampsia can present acutely without prior warning. **One third** of cases present for the **first time** post-delivery (usually in the first 48 hours). **The BP may only be mildly elevated at presentation** (i.e. 140/80–90 mmHg).

Eclampsia occurs in approximately 2.7:10,000 deliveries, usually beyond 24 weeks. It is one of the most dangerous complications of pregnancy, and is a significant cause of maternal mortality, with a mortality rate of 2% in the UK.

Convulsions are usually self-limiting but may be severe and repeated. The hypoxia caused during a tonic/clonic convulsion may lead to significant fetal compromise and death. An eclamptic fit is a **time critical** emergency for both the woman and the fetus.

Other complications associated with eclampsia include renal failure, hepatic failure and disseminated intravascular coagulation (DIC).

Risk factors include:
- known pre-eclampsia;
- primiparity or first child with a new partner;
- previous severe pre-eclampsia;
- essential hypertension;
- diabetes;

- obesity;
- twins or higher multiples;
- renal disease;
- advanced maternal age (over 35 years); and
- young maternal age (less than 16 years).

Assessment and management (Table 10.1):
- Undertake a primary survey – **ABCDEF** assessment.
- Assess for **time critical** features such as recurrent convulsions.

• If **non-time critical**, perform a more thorough assessment of the woman with secondary survey, including fetal assessment.	• **Note:** epileptic patients may suffer tonic/clonic convulsions. If > 20 weeks gestation with a history of hypertension or pre-eclampsia, treat as for eclampsia. • If there is no history of hypertension or pre-eclampsia and blood pressure is normal, treat as for epilepsy. • Protect the airway. Place the woman in a full lateral ('recovery') position – do not use the supine position with left lateral tilt. If formal resuscitation is required, use the supine position with manual uterine displacement (refer to Flowchart 7).
• Monitor SpO_2 (94–98%)	• Attach pulse oximeter; if SpO_2 < 94%, administer O_2 to aim for a target saturation within the range of 94–98%.

Table 10.1 Management of convulsions during pregnancy or after birth

• Continuous or recurrent convulsion	• If the patient convulses for longer than 2–3 minutes or has a second or subsequent convulsion, administer diazepam IV/PR titrated against effect (refer to any local policies on diazepam administration).
	Note: IV magnesium sulphate (4 grams slow IV over 10 minutes) can be given if available and avoids the use of multiple drugs.

Table 10.1 (*continued*)

Key Points for Convulsions During Pregnancy or After Birth

● Pregnancy-induced hypertension (PIH) and pre-eclampsia commonly occur beyond 24–28 weeks gestation but can occur as early as 22 weeks and up to 6 weeks post-delivery.

● A seizure in a pregnant woman should be considered eclampsia until proven otherwise.

● Diagnosis of pre-eclampsia includes an increase in blood pressure above 140/90 mmHg, oedema and detection of protein in the woman's urine.

● Eclampsia is one of the most dangerous complications of pregnancy. Involve the pre-hospital medical team early if it is difficult to manage the patient.

Chapter 10

Chapter 11

Special Considerations for Maternal Resuscitation

As outlined by the *Mother and Babies: Reducing Risk through Audits and Confidential Enquiries Across the UK: MBRRACE* report (Knight, 2015), 'for women in the United Kingdom, giving birth remains safer than ever – less than 9 in every 100,000 women die in pregnancy and around childbirth. Overall the maternal mortality rate in the UK continues to fall.'

Between 2012 and 2014, deaths from 'indirect' causes remain the most common; these are deaths from conditions not directly due to pregnancy but existing conditions which are exacerbated by pregnancy, for example women with heart problems. Given the very gradual rate of decline and the complexity of medical conditions now experienced by women during pregnancy, achieving the Government's ambition to reduce maternal deaths by 20% by 2020 and 50% by 2030 presents a major challenge for the health service that will require co-ordination of care across multiple specialities.

A maternal death is defined internationally as the death of a woman up to 6 weeks (42 days) after the end of pregnancy (whether the pregnancy ended by termination, miscarriage or a birth, or was an ectopic pregnancy) through causes associated with, or exacerbated by, pregnancy.

A late maternal death is one that occurs between 6 weeks and 1 year after the end of pregnancy.

Deaths are further subdivided on the basis of cause into:
- direct deaths, from pregnancy-specific causes, such as pre-eclampsia;
- indirect deaths, from other medical conditions made worse by pregnancy, such as cardiac disease; or
- coincidental deaths, where the cause is considered to be unrelated to pregnancy, such as road traffic accidents.

These definitions are summarised in Table 11.1.

• *Maternal death*	• The death of a woman while pregnant or within 42 days of the end of the pregnancy, including giving birth, ectopic pregnancy, miscarriage or termination of pregnancy, from any cause related to or aggravated by the pregnancy or its management, but not from accidental or incidental causes.
• *Direct death*	• Resulting from obstetric complications of the pregnant state (pregnancy, labour and puerperium), from interventions, omissions, incorrect treatment or from a chain of events resulting from any of the above.
• *Indirect death*	• Resulting from previous existing disease, or disease that developed during pregnancy and which was not the result of direct obstetric causes, but which was aggravated by the physiological effects of pregnancy.

Table 11.1 Categorisation and definitions of maternal deaths

• *Late death*	• Occurring between 42 days and 1 year after the end of pregnancy, including giving birth, ectopic pregnancy, miscarriage or termination of pregnancy, as the result of direct or indirect maternal causes.
• *Coincidental death*	• From unrelated causes that happen to occur in pregnancy or the puerperium. Termed 'fortuitous' in the International Classification of Diseases (ICD).

Table 11.1   (*continued*)

It is important to recognise that while there are two patients, resuscitation of the woman is the primary concern. Effective resuscitation of the woman may provide effective resuscitation of the fetus.

Request the pre-hospital medical team as early as possible where available.

If there is no response to CPR after 5 minutes, undertake a **time critical** transfer to the nearest ED with an obstetric unit attached. Place a pre-arrival information call as early as possible to enable the ED team to organise a maternity and neonatal team, as an immediate peri-mortem caesarean section (resuscitative hysterotomy) may be performed.

The approach to resuscitating a pregnant woman is the same as that of any adult in cardiac arrest. However, from 20 weeks gestation onwards, the weight of the gravid uterus can cause 30% of cardiac output to be sequestered into the lower limbs, with a woman lying supine.

Immediately manually displace the uterus to the maternal left side, relieving pressure on the inferior vena cava (refer to

Chapter 11

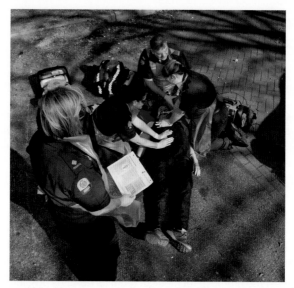

*Figure 11.1   Management of maternal cardiac arrest: manual uterine displacement from the maternal right side (**note lift and push**).*

Figure 11.1 and Figure 11.2). The action of uterine displacement may require the uterus to be lifted and either pushed over to the maternal left or lifted and pulled over to the maternal left depending upon the position of the person allocated to undertake the manoeuvre.

Manual uterine displacement should be continued throughout resuscitation, including when the woman is being conveyed to the hospital, as detailed in Figure 11.3.

CPR should not be terminated in the pre-hospital setting on a pregnant woman. While cardiac arrest in pregnancy is

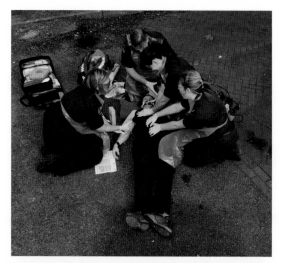

Figure 11.2 *Management of maternal cardiac arrest: manual uterine displacement from the maternal left side (**note lift and pull**).*

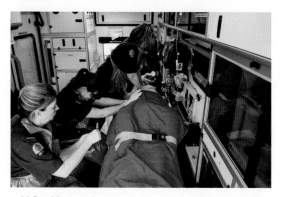

Figure 11.3 *Maternal resuscitation during transportation to hospital: manual uterine displacement is maintained.*

very rare, common causes of sudden maternal death include haemorrhage, embolism (thromboembolic and amniotic fluid) and hypertensive disorders. Table 11.2 details the reversible causes of maternal collapse.

Reversible cause		Cause in pregnancy
4Hs	Hypovolaemia	Bleeding (may be concealed) (obstetric/other) or relative hypovolaemia of dense spinal block; septic or neurogenic shock.
	Hypoxia	Pregnant women become hypoxic rapidly.
	Hypo/hyperkalaemia and other electrolyte disturbances	Cardiac events: peripartum cardiomyopathy, myocardial infarction, aortic dissection, large-vessel aneurysms.
	Hypothermia	No more likely.
4Ts	Thromboembolism	Amniotic fluid embolus, pulmonary embolus, air embolus, myocardial infarction.
	Toxicity	Local anaesthetic, magnesium, drug overdose, other.
	Tension pneumothorax	Following trauma/suicide attempt.
	Tamponade (cardiac)	Trauma
	Eclampsia and pre-eclampsia	Includes intracranial haemorrhage.

Table 11.2 Causes of maternal collapse

Management of Maternal Cardiac Arrest

Commence resuscitation according to standard ALS guidance with manual uterine displacement to the maternal left to minimise inferior vena caval compression. The hand position for chest compressions may need to be slightly higher (2–3 cm) on the sternum for women in advanced pregnancy (e.g. more than 28 weeks).

Where the skill set is available, intubate early. Consider using a tracheal tube 0.5–1.0 mm smaller than usual as the trachea can be narrowed by oedema and swelling. Supraglottic airway devices are a suitable alternative in the pre-hospital setting and may provide a more rapid means of oxygenation than potentially prolonged intubation attempts.

Defibrillation energy levels are as recommended for standard defibrillation. If large breasts make it difficult to place an apical defibrillator electrode, use an anterior–posterior or bi-axillary electrode position.

Establish intravenous or intraosseous access as soon as possible, preferably at a level above the diaphragm.

Where possible, identify and correct the cause of the cardiac arrest using the 4Hs and 4Ts, as per Table 11.1.

Oxygen should be administered as soon as available.

Undertake a **time critical** transfer to the nearest ED with an obstetric unit, or ED. A pre-arrival information call should be placed as early as possible to enable the ED team to organise a maternity team.

The Team Approach to Pre-hospital Resuscitation (Resuscitation Council, 2015)

Resuscitation requires a system to be in place to achieve the best possible chance of survival. The system requires technical and non-technical skills (teamwork, situational awareness, leadership, decision making) in the assessment and management of the pregnant woman. This will also involve consideration for manual uterine displacement.

Allocation of roles:

• Appoint a team leader as early as possible, ideally a paramedic or clinician experienced in pre-hospital resuscitation.

• The team leader should assign team members specific roles, which they clearly understand and are capable of undertaking. This will promote teamwork, reduce confusion and ensure organised and effective management of resuscitation.

• A minimum of four trained staff is required to deliver high quality resuscitation. This will necessitate dispatch of more than one ambulance resource.

• Ensure there is 360° access to the patient ('Circle of Life'), as in Figure 11.1:

○ Position 1: Airway (at head of patient) – the person must be trained and equipped to provide the full range of airway skills.

○ Position 2: High-quality chest compressions and defibrillation if needed – at patient's left side. Be prepared to alternate with the operator at position 3 to avoid fatigue.

○ Position 3: High-quality chest compressions and access to the circulation (intravenous, intraosseous) – at patient's right side.

○ Position 4: Team leader – stands back and oversees the resuscitation attempt, only becoming involved if required. The team leader should have an awareness of the whole incident and ensure high-quality resuscitation is maintained and appropriate decisions made.

The team leader will need to allocate the role of manual uterine displacement and may necessitate the involvement of additional resources where available.

Key Points for Maternal Resuscitation

- Request a pre-hospital team where available, as early as possible. **Always** manage pregnant women in cardiac arrest at greater than 20 weeks gestation with manual displacement of the uterus to the maternal left.

- If resuscitation attempts fail to achieve a return of spontaneous circulation within 5 minutes of the cardiac arrest, undertake a **time critical** transfer to the nearest ED with an obstetric unit attached.

- Provide an early pre-arrival information call detailing '**maternal cardiac arrest**' to enable the ED to summon the maternity and neonatal team as an immediate peri-mortem caesarean section (resuscitative hysterotomy) may be performed.

Chapter 11

Chapter 12

Special Considerations for Newborn Resuscitation

Passage through the birth canal is a hypoxic event for the fetus, since placental respiratory exchange is prevented for the 50–75 seconds duration of the average contraction. Most babies tolerate this well and are able to make the transition to normal breathing within a minute of birth, but for those few who do not, help will be required to establish normal breathing.

The newborn life support guideline outlines this help and comprises the following elements:
* drying and covering the baby to conserve heat;
* assessing the need for any intervention;
* opening the airway;
* lung aeration;
* ventilation breaths; and
* chest compressions.

In the face of in-utero hypoxia, the breathing centre in the fetal brain becomes depressed and spontaneous breathing movement ceases. The fetus can maintain an effective circulation during periods of hypoxia, so the most urgent requirement for a hypoxic baby at birth is aeration of the lungs. Provided the circulation has remained intact, oxygenated blood will be conveyed from the lungs to the heart and onwards to the brain. The breathing centre should then recover and the baby will breathe spontaneously.

Babies are born wet and can become cold very easily, particularly if they remain wet and exposed. Dry the baby, paying particular attention to the head, apply a newborn hat if available and cover the baby with a dry towel. A baby that does not require resuscitation should be placed with the mother, providing skin-to-skin contact. This will afford the opportunity for early feeding and reduce the risk of hypoglycaemia. Make continuous observations of the baby's airway position and breathing. For pre-term babies who are breathing and do not require resuscitation, they too should be placed skin-to-skin with the mother. Foil cribs or heating mattresses may afford benefits in this group of babies to optimise body temperature.

A temperature must be recorded as soon as practicable after birth and repeated during transport.
- A healthy baby will be born blue but will have a good tone and will breathe spontaneously within a minute of birth. In a healthy term baby, the heart rate is greater than 100 bpm by 2 minutes of age and it will become pink within the first minute or two.
- A less healthy baby will be born blue, will have reduced tone, may have a slow heart rate (60–100 bpm) and may not establish adequate breathing by 2 minutes.
- An ill (very hypoxic) baby will be born pale and floppy, not breathing and with a very slow heart rate (less than 60 bpm).

In all cases, ensure the ambient temperature is around 25°, and close windows and doors to reduce draughts.

Position the baby where there is 360° access to enable management of the airway and chest in case further intervention is required.

Dry the baby from head to toe while completing **ABC** assessment. If available apply a newborn hat and wrap in a new, warm, dry towel. Avoid covering the face and airway. Delay clamping and cutting the umbilical cord unless resuscitation is required.

Assess the colour, tone, breathing and heart rate of the baby.
- Assess heart rate by listening with a stethoscope (feeling for a peripheral pulse is not reliable).
- In noisy or very cold environments, palpating the pulse at the umbilical cord may be an alternative and may save unwrapping the baby (this is only reliable when the pulse is more than 100 bpm).
- If available attach a pulse oximeter (placed on the right wrist, this can provide an accurate heart rate in approximately 90 seconds and provide an accurate oxygen saturation).

Re-assess breathing and heart rate every 30 seconds. An increase in heart rate is usually the first clinical sign of improvement.

Decide whether help is required (and likely to be available) and whether rapid transfer to hospital is indicated.
- Ensure the heat in the transport is set to maximum.
- Once the baby is being transferred, continue to monitor its condition and maintain the temperature en route.

Airway:
- Place the baby on its back, with the head in the neutral position, neither flexed nor extended (Figure 12.1).
- If the baby is very floppy, a chin lift or jaw thrust may be required.
- A small pad (2 cm) can be placed under the shoulders to assist in maintaining the neutral position (Figure 12.2).

Breathing:
- Give 5 inflation breaths, sustaining the inflation pressure at about 30 cm of water for 2–3 seconds with each breath – use a 500 ml bag-valve-mask device.
- The first two or three breaths replace the fluid in the lungs with air without changing the volume in the chest. Therefore, you may not observe the chest wall rise until the fourth or fifth breath.

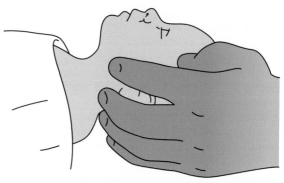

Figure 12.1   Neutral position.

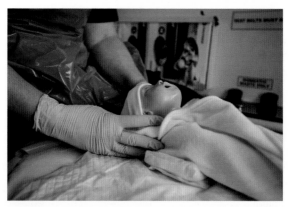

Figure 12.2   Neutral position with pad under shoulders.

Heart rate:
- If the heart rate increases, assume that lung aeration has been successful.
- If the heart rate increases but the baby **does not start breathing**:

  ○ Continue to provide regular breaths (ventilation breaths) at a rate of about 30–40 per minute until the baby starts to breathe on their own.

  ○ Note: Ventilation breaths are given at a rate of one every two seconds; the aim is to establish 30–40 per minute. Continue to monitor the heart rate. If the rate should drop to < 100 bpm it suggests insufficient ventilation. In this situation, increase the rate of inflation or use a longer inspiratory time.

- If the heart rate does not increase following inflation breaths:

  ○ Either lung aeration has not been adequate or the baby requires more than lung aeration alone.

  ○ It is most likely that you have not aerated the lungs effectively. Repeat the procedure of inflation breaths.

  ○ Note: If the heart rate does not increase and the chest does not move with each inflation, you have not aerated the lungs; in this situation consider:

    – Is the head in the neutral position?

    – Do you need to do a jaw thrust?

    – Do you need a longer inflation time?

    – Do you need help with the airway from a second person?

    – Is there obstruction in the oropharynx? Where an appropriately sized laryngoscope is available, it may be used to inspect the airway and remove any obvious obstructions, where the clinician has the expertise.

    – Do you need an oropharyngeal airway?

- If after a further set of 5 inflation breaths and 30 seconds of ventilation breaths the heart rate remains less than 60 bpm, or the heart beat is absent **despite** chest wall rise:

  ○ Commence chest compressions ensuring the baby is on a flat, hard surface (not a mattress or sofa), see Figure 12.3.

  ○ Encircle the lower chest with both hands in such a way that the two thumbs can compress the lower third of the sternum, at a point just below an imaginary line joining the nipples, with the fingers over the spine at the back.

○ Compress the chest quickly and firmly in such a way as to reduce the anterior–posterior diameter of the chest by a third.
○ The ratio of compressions to inflations in newborn resuscitation is 3:1.
○ Compress at a rate of 120 compressions per minute i.e. approximately 90 compressions and 30 ventilations.
○ ECG complexes do not indicate the presence of a cardiac output and should not be the sole means of monitoring the infant. However, improving heart rate on ECG is likely to indicate successful ventilation and some cardiac output.
○ If the baby does not respond very rapidly to bag-valve-mask ventilation and cardiac compressions, undertake a **time critical** transfer.
○ Provide a pre-arrival information call detailing '**newborn resuscitation**' and convey to the nearest ED with an obstetric unit or medical facility.

Meconium:
● Attempting to aspirate meconium from a baby's mouth and nose while their head is still on the perineum does not prevent meconium aspiration and is **not** recommended.
● Attempting to aspirate meconium from a vigorous baby's airway after birth will not prevent meconium aspiration and is **not** recommended (this may induce a vagal response in the baby and cause bradycardia).
● If a baby is born through thick meconium and is unresponsive at birth, the oropharynx must be inspected and cleared of meconium first. The focus should be on inflating the lungs, and the trachea should only be suctioned if a suitable laryngoscope and the expertise is available and the trachea is thought to be blocked. Attempts at lung inflation and ventilation must not be unduly delayed.

Special considerations:
● Commence resuscitation with air. Introduce supplemental oxygen if there is not a rapid improvement in the baby's condition and compressions are required.

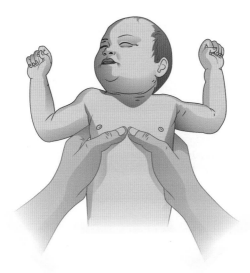

Figure 12.3 *Newborn chest compressions.*

● For uncompromised term and pre-term infants, delay cord clamping at least 2 minutes from the complete delivery of the infant and until the cord stops pulsating.

Key Points for Newborn Resuscitation

● Passage through the birth canal is a hypoxic event and some babies may require help to establish normal breathing after birth.

● Ensure the airway is open by placing the baby on its back with the head in a neutral position.

● If the baby is not breathing adequately within 60 seconds, give five inflation breaths.

● If chest compressions are necessary, compress the chest quickly and firmly at a ratio of 3:1 compressions to inflations using a two-thumbs encircling technique.

Flowchart 1: Normal Birth

UNDERTAKE PRIMARY SURVEY
Establish gestation and frequency of contractions

↓

BIRTH IMMINENT

↓

Request midwife if available
Prepare for newborn life support
Reassure the woman and support her in a
comfortable position, avoiding the supine position
Provide Entonox for pain relief

↓

Support the birth of the baby's head by
applying gentle pressure as the head advances

↓

Support the baby during the birth and
place on the maternal abdomen

↓

Thoroughly dry the baby with a warm
towel and wrap with a dry towel

↓

If the baby is crying, provide
'skin-to-skin' contact with the mother

↓

Allow the umbilical cord to stop
pulsating prior to clamping and cutting

↓

The placenta may take 15–20 mins to birth – **DO NOT**
pull on the cord – encourage the mother to pass urine

Deliver the placenta into a plastic bag for the midwife
to inspect and check for completeness

Assess and record estimated blood loss

If the placenta remains undelivered with minimal
bleeding, plan to transfer to the nearest appropriate
destination as agreed locally

Maternal safety is the prime consideration

Consider the specific clinical situation **and which
interventions may be required for the woman
and baby on arrival**

Refer to 'Appropriate Destination for Conveyance'
in **Chapter 1.**

If the placenta remains undelivered and bleeding,
refer to **Flowchart 5: Post-partum Haemorrhage**

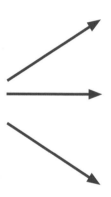

Flowcharts

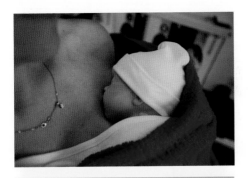

If the baby is not crying refer to

Flowchart 8: Newborn Resuscitation

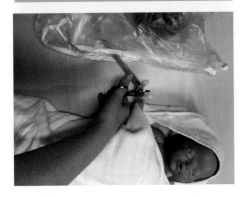

Flowchart 2: Cord Prolapse

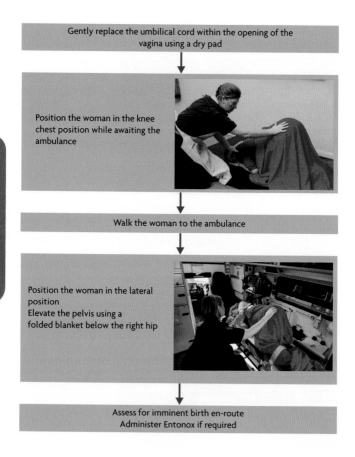

Gently replace the umbilical cord within the opening of the vagina using a dry pad

⬇

Position the woman in the knee chest position while awaiting the ambulance

⬇

Walk the woman to the ambulance

⬇

Position the woman in the lateral position
Elevate the pelvis using a folded blanket below the right hip

⬇

Assess for imminent birth en-route
Administer Entonox if required

Transfer to nearest appropriate destination as agreed locally
Maternal safety is the prime consideration
Consider the specific clinical situation **and which interventions may be required for the woman and baby on arrival**
Refer to 'Appropriate Destination for Conveyance' in **Chapter 1**
Pre-alert stating obstetric emergency of cord prolapse
Take maternity notes if available

Flowchart 3: Breech Birth

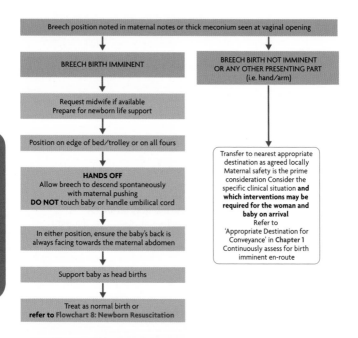

Breech position noted in maternal notes or thick meconium seen at vaginal opening

BREECH BIRTH IMMINENT

BREECH BIRTH NOT IMMINENT OR ANY OTHER PRESENTING PART
(i.e. hand/arm)

Request midwife if available
Prepare for newborn life support

Position on edge of bed/trolley or on all fours

HANDS OFF
Allow breech to descend spontaneously with maternal pushing
DO NOT touch baby or handle umbilical cord

In either position, ensure the baby's back is always facing towards the maternal abdomen

Support baby as head births

Treat as normal birth or
refer to Flowchart 8: Newborn Resuscitation

Transfer to nearest appropriate destination as agreed locally Maternal safety is the prime consideration Consider the specific clinical situation **and which interventions may be required for the woman and baby on arrival** Refer to 'Appropriate Destination for Conveyance' in **Chapter 1** Continuously assess for birth imminent en-route

IF DELAY OCCURS DURING THE BIRTH:

LEGS: apply gentle pressure behind the baby's knee
ARMS: gently rotate the baby's pelvis 90 degrees to aid birth of the first arm – rotate the baby's body in the opposite direction if required to birth the second arm – allow the baby's body to hang unassisted
HEAD: support the baby with one arm and use the other hand to aid flexion of the back of the baby's head while delivering baby

DO NOT PULL ON THE BABY
DO NOT CLAMP AND CUT THE UMBILICAL CORD DURING THE BIRTH

Flowcharts

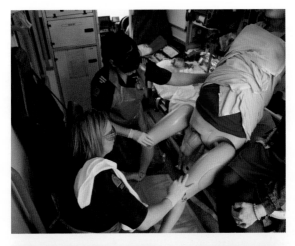

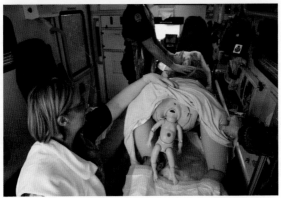

Flowchart 4: Shoulder Dystocia

REQUEST A MIDWIFE IF AVAILABLE AND PREPARE FOR NEWBORN LIFE SUPPORT
Position the woman in the McRoberts position
For a solo clinician – ask the woman to hold her legs and push with her next contraction

If shoulders do not release:
Attempt to deliver the baby
- With your hands on the baby's head apply gentle 'axial' traction, keeping the baby's head in line with its spine for up to 30 seconds

Undelivered?

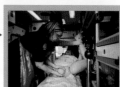

Apply suprapubic pressure with the woman in the McRoberts position
- Identify the position of the fetal back and place assistant on that maternal side
- Using a CPR grip, apply continuous pressure downwards and lateral for 30 seconds (2 fingers above symphysis pubis)
- Encourage the woman to push **OR** attempt gentle 'axial' traction to deliver baby

Undelivered?

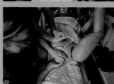

- Attempt intermittent 'rocking' suprapubic pressure for 30 seconds and encourage woman to push
- Or attempt gentle 'axial' traction to deliver baby

Undelivered?

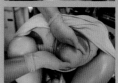

- Change the woman's position to 'all fours' and encourage her to push
- Or attempt gentle 'axial' traction to deliver baby

Undelivered?

- Walk the woman to the ambulance and anticipate the birth during transfer
- Convey in a lateral position with legs separated by a blanket to protect the baby's head
- Reassure the woman and provide Entonox as required

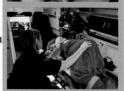

Baby born

Flowchart 5: Post-partum Haemorrhage

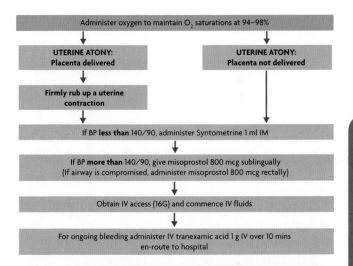

Administer oxygen to maintain O₂ saturations at 94–98%

UTERINE ATONY:
Placenta delivered

UTERINE ATONY:
Placenta not delivered

Firmly rub up a uterine contraction

If BP **less than** 140/90, administer Syntometrine 1 ml IM

If BP **more than** 140/90, give misoprostol 800 mcg sublingually
(If airway is compromised, administer misoprostol 800 mcg rectally)

Obtain IV access (16G) and commence IV fluids

For ongoing bleeding administer IV tranexamic acid 1 g IV over 10 mins
en-route to hospital

If uterus is well contracted, check for perineal trauma:
Apply external direct pressure gauze/maternity pad
Obtain IV access (16G) and commence IV fluids
For ongoing bleeding administer IV tranexamic acid 1 g IV over 10 mins
en-route to hospital

Transfer to nearest appropriate destination as agreed locally
Maternal safety is the prime consideration
Consider the specific clinical situation **and which interventions may be**
required for the woman and baby on arrival
Refer to 'Appropriate Destination for Conveyance' in **Chapter 1**
Pre-alert stating obstetric emergency PPH
Perform ongoing assessment of uterine contraction
and/or perineal trauma/maternal observations

Flowchart 6: Convulsions in Pregnancy and After Birth

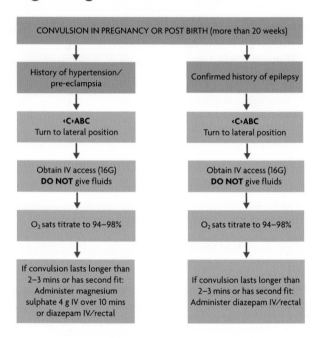

CONVULSION IN PREGNANCY OR POST BIRTH (more than 20 weeks)

History of hypertension/ pre-eclampsia	Confirmed history of epilepsy
‹C›ABC Turn to lateral position	‹C›ABC Turn to lateral position
Obtain IV access (16G) **DO NOT** give fluids	Obtain IV access (16G) **DO NOT** give fluids
O₂ sats titrate to 94–98%	O₂ sats titrate to 94–98%
If convulsion lasts longer than 2–3 mins or has second fit: Administer magnesium sulphate 4 g IV over 10 mins or diazepam IV/rectal	If convulsion lasts longer than 2–3 mins or has second fit: Administer diazepam IV/rectal

Transfer to nearest appropriate destination as agreed locally
Maternal safety is the prime consideration
Consider the specific clinical situation **and which
interventions may be required for the woman
and baby on arrival**
Refer to 'Appropriate Destination for Conveyance'
in **Chapter 1**
Pre-alert stating obstetric emergency eclampsia
Take maternity notes if available

Flowchart 7: Maternal Resuscitation

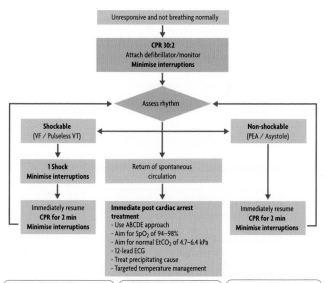

Unresponsive and not breathing normally

CPR 30:2
Attach defibrillator/monitor
Minimise interruptions

Assess rhythm

Shockable
(VF / Pulseless VT)

Non-shockable
(PEA / Asystole)

1 Shock
Minimise interruptions

Return of spontaneous circulation

Immediately resume
CPR for 2 min
Minimise interruptions

Immediate post cardiac arrest treatment
- Use ABCDE approach
- Aim for SpO$_2$ of 94–98%
- Aim for normal EtCO$_2$ of 4.7–6.4 kPa
- 12-lead ECG
- Treat precipitating cause
- Targeted temperature management

Immediately resume
CPR for 2 min
Minimise interruptions

DURING CPR	TREAT REVERSIBLE CAUSES	CONSIDER
• If pregnancy > 20 weeks, manually displace uterus to maternal left. • Ensure high-quality chest compressions. • Minimise interruptions to compressions. • Give oxygen. • Use waveform capnography. • Continuous compressions when advanced airway in place. • Vascular access (intravenous or intraosseous). • Give adrenaline every 3–5 min. • Give amiodarone after 3 shocks.	• **H**ypoxia. • **H**ypovolaemia. • **H**ypo/hyperkalaemia/metabolic. • **H**ypothermia. • **T**hrombosis – coronary or pulmonary. • **T**ension pneumothorax. • **T**amponade – cardiac. • **T**oxins. • Eclampsia. • Pre-eclampsia.	• Failure to get ROSC in 5 minutes, take to the nearest emergency department. • Ultrasound imaging. • Follow local protocols for chest compressions. Where available consider mechanical chest compressions. • Transfer for coronary angiography and percutaneous coronary intervention.

Flowcharts

Flowchart 8: Newborn Resuscitation

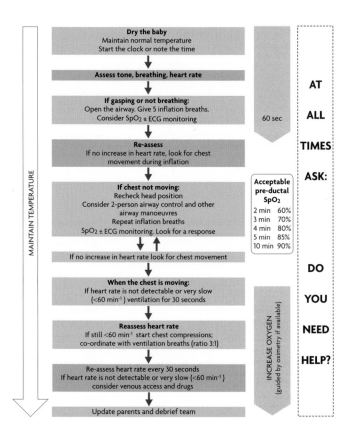

Dry the baby
Maintain normal temperature
Start the clock or note the time

↓

Assess tone, breathing, heart rate

↓

If gasping or not breathing:
Open the airway. Give 5 inflation breaths.
Consider SpO₂ ± ECG monitoring

↓

Re-assess
If no increase in heart rate, look for chest
movement during inflation

↓

If chest not moving:
Recheck head position
Consider 2-person airway control and other
airway manoeuvres
Repeat inflation breaths
SpO₂ ± ECG monitoring. Look for a response

↓

If no increase in heart rate look for chest movement

↓

When the chest is moving:
If heart rate is not detectable or very slow
(<60 min⁻¹) ventilation for 30 seconds

↓

Reassess heart rate
If still <60 min⁻¹ start chest compressions;
co-ordinate with ventilation breaths (ratio 3:1)

↓

Re-assess heart rate every 30 seconds
If heart rate is not detectable or very slow (<60 min⁻¹)
consider venous access and drugs

↓

Update parents and debrief team

MAINTAIN TEMPERATURE

60 sec

Acceptable pre-ductal SpO₂	
2 min	60%
3 min	70%
4 min	80%
5 min	85%
10 min	90%

INCREASE OXYGEN (guided by oximetry if available)

AT ALL TIMES ASK:

DO YOU NEED HELP?

Flowcharts

82

APGAR Score

	0	1	2	
Appearance	Blue or pale all over	Blue at extremities Body pink	Body and extremities pink	
Pulse rate	Absent	<100	≥100	
Grimace or response to stimulation	No response to simulation	Grimace/ feeble cry when stimulated	Cry or pull away when stimulated	
Activity or muscle tone	None	Some flexion	Flexed arms and legs that resist extension	
Respiration	Absent	Weak, irregular, gasping	Strong, lusty cry	
Total score		+	+	=

Birth Summary Card 1: Mother

Time of birth of the head

Time of birth

Cephalic birth

Breech Birth

Multiple birth

Location of birth

Birth Summary Card 2: Baby

Records

Date of birth

Time of birth

Sex   M / F

Gestation at birth

Skin to skin

Newborn Comments

Meconium present

Breech Birth

Shoulder Dystocia

Summary

Bibliography and Further Reading

Maternity Care, Assessment of the Pregnant Woman, Emergency Birth and Newborn Care

1. Beard L, Lax P and Tindall M. (2016) Physiological effects of transfer for critically ill patients. *Anaesthesia Tutorial of the Week*, 330. Available at: http://anaesthesiology.gr/media/File/pdf/330-Physiological-effects-of-transfer-for-critically-ill-patients.pdf.

2. Bourjeily G, Paidas M, Khalil H, et al. (2010) Pulmonary embolism in pregnancy. *The Lancet*, 375(9713): 500–512.

3. Catchpole. (2010) cited in Department of Health. (2012) *Human Factors Reference Group Interim Report, 1 March 2012*. National Quality Board. Available at: http://www.england.nhs.uk/ourwork/part-rel/nqb/ag-min/.

4. Centre for Maternal and Child Enquiries. (2011) Saving mothers' lives: reviewing maternal deaths to make motherhood safer: 2006–2008. *BJOG: An International Journal of Obstetrics & Gynaecology*, 118 (suppl. 1).

5. Cornblath M, Hawdon JM, Williams AF, et al. (2000) Controversies regarding definition of neonatal hypoglycemia: suggested operational thresholds. *Pediatrics*, 105(5): 1141–1145.

6. Crofts JF, Lenguerrand E, Bentham GL, et al. (2016) Prevention of brachial plexus injury – 12 years of shoulder dystocia training: an interrupted time-series study. *BJOG: An International Journal of Obstetrics & Gynaecology*, 123(1): 111–118.

7. Gherman RB. (2016) Shoulder dystocia. *Clinical Obstetrics and Gynecology*, 59(4): 789–790.

8. Griffin C. (2016) Re: Prevention of brachial plexus injury – 12 years of shoulder dystocia training: an interrupted time-series study: posterior arm delivery at the time of caesarean section. *BJOG: An International Journal of Obstetrics & Gynaecology*, 123(1): 144.

9. Hawdon JM. (2012) Investigation, prevention and management of neonatal hypoglycaemia (impaired postnatal metabolic adaptation). *Paediatrics and Child Health*, 22(4): 131–135.

10. Health and Care Professions Council. (2003) *Standards of Conduct, Performance and Ethics: Your Duties as a Registrant*. London: Health Professions Council.

11. Knight M, Tuffnell D, Kenyon S, et al. (eds) on behalf of MBRRACE-UK. (2015) *Saving Lives, Improving Mothers' Care – Surveillance of maternal deaths in the UK 2011–13 and lessons learned to inform maternity care from the UK and Ireland Confidential Enquiries into Maternal Deaths and Morbidity 2009–13*. Oxford: National Perinatal Epidemiology Unit, University of Oxford.

12. Menticoglou S. (2016) Delivering shoulders and dealing with shoulder dystocia: should the standard of care change? *Journal of Obstetrics and Gynaecology Canada*, 38(7): 655–658.

13. Mousa HA and Alfirevic Z. (2007) Treatment for primary postpartum haemorrhage. *Cochrane Database of Systematic Reviews*, 1: CD003249.

14. National Collaborating Centre for Women's and Children's Health. (2008) *Diabetes in Pregnancy* (CG63). London: National Institute for Health and Clinical Excellence.

15. National Institute for Health and Clinical Excellence. (2010) *Neonatal Jaundice: Treatment Threshold Graphs*. London: NICE. Available at: https://www.nice.org.uk/guidance/cg98/evidence/full-guideline-pdf-245411821.

16. Porter A, Snooks H, Youren A, et al. (2008) 'Covering our backs': ambulance crews' attitudes towards clinical documentation when emergency (999) patients are not conveyed to hospital. *Emergency Medicine Journal*, 25(5): 292–295.

17. Royal College of Obstetricians and Gynaecologists. (2006) *The Management of Breech Presentation* (Green-top Guideline 20b). London: RCOG.

18. Royal College of Obstetricians and Gynaecologists. (2008) *Umbilical Cord Prolapse* (Green-top Guideline 50). London: RCOG.

19. Royal College of Obstetricians and Gynaecologists. (2011) *Placenta Praevia, Placenta Praevia Accreta and Vasa Praevia: Diagnosis and Management* (Green-top Guideline 27). London: RCOG.

20. Royal College of Obstetricians and Gynaecologists. (2012) *Shoulder Dystocia* (Green-top Guideline 42). London RCOG.

21. Royal College of Obstetricians and Gynaecologists. (2016) *Prevention and Management of Postpartum Haemorrhage* (Green-top Guideline 52). London: RCOG.

22. Starrs A and Winikoff B. (2012) Misoprostol for postpartum hemorrhage: moving from evidence to practice. *International Journal of Gynaecology and Obstetrics*, 116(1): 1–3.

23. Woollard M, Hinshaw K, Simpson H and Wieteska S. (2009) Care of the baby at birth. In *Pre-hospital Obstetric Emergency Training*. Oxford: Wiley-Blackwell: 125–135.

24. Woollard M, Hinshaw K, Simpson H and Wieteska S. (2009) Emergencies after delivery. In *Pre-hospital Obstetric Emergency Training*. Oxford: Wiley-Blackwell: 111–124.

25. Woollard M, Hinshaw K, Simpson H and Wieteska S. (2009) Emergencies in late pregnancy. In *Pre-hospital Obstetric Emergency Training*. Oxford: Wiley-Blackwell: 62–110.

26. Woollard M, Hinshaw K, Simpson H and Wieteska S. (2009) Normal delivery. In *Pre-hospital Obstetric Emergency Training*. Oxford: Wiley-Blackwell: 28–37.

27. Woollard M, Hinshaw K, Simpson H and Wieteska S (eds). (2009) *Pre-hospital Obstetric Emergency Training*. Oxford: Wiley-Blackwell.

28. Woollard M, Hinshaw K, Simpson H and Wieteska S. (2009) Structured approach to the obstetric patient. In *Pre-hospital Obstetric Emergency Training*. Oxford: Wiley-Blackwell: 38–52.

29. Wyllie J, Bruinenberg J, Roehr CC, et al. (2015) European Resuscitation Council Guidelines for Resuscitation 2015. Section 7: Resuscitation and support of transition of babies at birth. *Resuscitation*, 95: 249–263.

30. Wyllie J, Perlman JM, Kattwinkel J, et al. (2010) Part 11: Neonatal resuscitation: 2010 International Consensus on Cardiopulmonary Resuscitation and Emergency Cardiovascular Care Science with Treatment Recommendations. *Resuscitation*, 81(1): e260–287.

31. Wyllie J, Perlman JM, Kattwinkel J, et al. (2015) Part 7: Neonatal resuscitation: 2015 International Consensus on Cardiopulmonary Resuscitation and Emergency Cardiovascular Care Science with Treatment Recommendations. *Resuscitation*, 95: e169–201.

Bleeding in Pregnancy

1. Human Tissue Authority. (2015) *Guidance on the Disposal of Pregnancy Remains Following Pregnancy Loss or Termination*.

Available at: https://www.hta.gov.uk/sites/default/files/Guidance_
on_the_disposal_of_pregnancy_remains.pdf.

2. Royal College of Nursing. (2015) *Managing the Disposal of
Pregnancy Remains. RCN Guidance for Nursing and Midwifery
Practice*. Available at: https://www2.rcn.org.uk/__data/assets/pdf_
file/0008/645884/RCNguide_disposal_pregnancy_remains_WEB.
pdf.

3. Soar J, Perkins GD, Abbas G, et al. (2010) European Resuscitation
Council Guidelines for Resuscitation 2010. Section 8: Cardiac
arrest in special circumstances: electrolyte abnormalities,
poisoning, drowning, accidental hypothermia, hyperthermia,
asthma, anaphylaxis, cardiac surgery, trauma, pregnancy,
electrocution. *Resuscitation*, 81(10): 1400–1433.

4. Woollard M, Hinshaw K, Simpson H and Wieteska S. (2009)
Anatomical and physiological changes in pregnancy. In *Pre-hospital
Obstetric Emergency Training*. Oxford: Wiley-Blackwell: 18–27.

5. Woollard M, Hinshaw K, Simpson H and Wieteska S. (2009)
Emergencies in early pregnancy and complications following
gynaecological surgery. In *Pre-hospital Obstetric Emergency
Training*. Oxford: Wiley-Blackwell: 53–61.

6. Woollard M, Hinshaw K, Simpson H and Wieteska S. (2009)
Emergencies in late pregnancy. In *Pre-hospital Obstetric
Emergency Training*. Oxford: Wiley-Blackwell: 62–110.

7. Woollard M, Hinshaw K, Simpson H and Wieteska S. (2009)
Obstetric services. In *Pre-hospital Obstetric Emergency Training*.
Oxford: Wiley-Blackwell: 1–6.

8. Woollard M, Hinshaw K, Simpson H and Wieteska S. (2009)
Structured approach to the obstetric patient. In *Pre-hospital
Obstetric Emergency Training*. Oxford: Wiley-Blackwell: 38–52.

Convulsions During Pregnancy or After Birth

1. Centre for Maternal and Child Enquiries. (2011) Saving mothers'
lives: reviewing maternal deaths to make motherhood safer:
2006–2008. *BJOG: An International Journal of Obstetrics &
Gynaecology*, 118(suppl. 1).

2. Soar J, Perkins GD, Abbas G, et al. (2010) European Resuscitation
Council Guidelines for Resuscitation 2010. Section 8: Cardiac

arrest in special circumstances: electrolyte abnormalities, poisoning, drowning, accidental hypothermia, hyperthermia, asthma, anaphylaxis, cardiac surgery, trauma, pregnancy, electrocution. *Resuscitation*, 81(10): 1400–1433.

3. Woollard M, Hinshaw K, Simpson H and Wieteska S. (2009) Anatomical and physiological changes in pregnancy. In *Pre-hospital Obstetric Emergency Training*. Oxford: Wiley-Blackwell: 18–27.

4. Woollard M, Hinshaw K, Simpson H and Wieteska S. (2009) Emergencies in late pregnancy. In *Pre-hospital Obstetric Emergency Training*. Oxford: Wiley-Blackwell: 62–110.

5. Woollard M, Hinshaw K, Simpson H and Wieteska S. (2009) Obstetric services. In *Pre-hospital Obstetric Emergency Training*. Oxford: Wiley-Blackwell: 1–6.

6. Woollard M, Hinshaw K, Simpson H and Wieteska S. (2009) Structured approach to the obstetric patient. In *Pre-hospital Obstetric Emergency Training*. Oxford: Wiley-Blackwell: 38–52.

Special Considerations for Maternal Resuscitation

1. Deakin CD, Nolan JP, Soar J, et al. (2010) European Resuscitation Council Guidelines for Resuscitation 2010. Section 4: Adult advanced life support. *Resuscitation*, 81(10): 1305–1352.

2. Deakin CD, Nolan JP, Sunde K and Koster RW. (2010) European Resuscitation Council Guidelines for Resuscitation 2010. Section 3: Electrical therapies: automated external defibrillators, defibrillation, cardioversion and pacing. *Resuscitation*, 81(10): 1293–1304.

3. Knight M, Tuffnell D, Kenyon S, et al. (eds) on behalf of MBRRACE-UK. (2015) *Saving Lives, Improving Mothers' Care – Surveillance of maternal deaths in the UK 2011–13 and lessons learned to inform maternity care from the UK and Ireland Confidential Enquiries into Maternal Deaths and Morbidity 2009–13*. Oxford: National Perinatal Epidemiology Unit, University of Oxford.

4. Koster RW, Baubin MA, Bossaert LL, et al. (2010) European Resuscitation Council Guidelines for Resuscitation 2010. Section

2: Adult basic life support and use of automated external defibrillators. *Resuscitation*, 81(10): 1277–1292.

5. Resuscitation Council. (2015) Prehospital resuscitation. Available at: https://www.resus.org.uk/resuscitation-guidelines/prehospital-resuscitation.

6. Royal College of Obstetricians and Gynaecologists. (2010, updated 2014) *Maternal Collapse in Pregnancy and the Puerperium* (Green-top Guideline 56). London: RCOG. Available at: https://www.rcog.org.uk/globalassets/documents/guidelines/gtg_56.pdf.

7. Soar J, Perkins GD, Abbas G, et al. (2010) European Resuscitation Council Guidelines for Resuscitation 2010. Section 8: Cardiac arrest in special circumstances: electrolyte abnormalities, poisoning, drowning, accidental hypothermia, hyperthermia, asthma, anaphylaxis, cardiac surgery, trauma, pregnancy, electrocution. *Resuscitation*, 81(10): 1400–1433.

8. World Health Organization. (2010) International Classification of Diseases (ICD) 10. Available at: http://www.who.int/classifications/icd/en/.

Special Considerations for Newborn Resuscitation

1. Belsches TC, Tilly AE, Miller TR, et al. (2013) Randomised trial of plastic bags to prevent term neonatal hypothermia in a resource-poor setting. *Pediatrics*, 132(3). Available at: http://pediatrics.aappublications.org/content/132/3/e656.

2. Leadford AE, Warren JB, Manasyan A, et al. (2013) Plastic bags for prevention of hypothermia in preterm and low birth weight infants. *Pediatrics*, 132(1). Available at: http://pediatrics.aappublications.org/content/132/1/e128.

3. Wyllie J, Bruinenberg J, Roehr CC, et al. (2015) European Resuscitation Council Guidelines for Resuscitation 2015. Section 7. Resuscitation and support of transition of babies at birth. *Resuscitation*, 95: 249–263.

4. Wyllie J, Perlman JM, Kattwinkel J, et al. (2015) Part 7: Neonatal resuscitation: 2015 International Consensus on Cardiopulmonary Resuscitation and Emergency Cardiovascular Care Science with Treatment Recommendations. *Resuscitation*, 95: e169–201.

Index

Index

Index

Notes

Notes

Notes

Notes

Notes

Notes

Notes

Notes